FASTING FORWARD

A journey away from
addiction to food

Zachary Scott Turnage

Kindle Direct Publishing

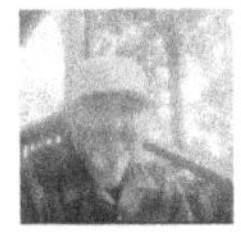

ISBN: 9798320813059 hardcover

ISBN: 9798320797793 paperback

Cover design by: Art Painter
Library of Congress Control Number: 2018675309
Printed in the United States of America

*I dedicate this book to my beautiful
Daughter (Kaylie Dakota Turnage)*

CONTENTS

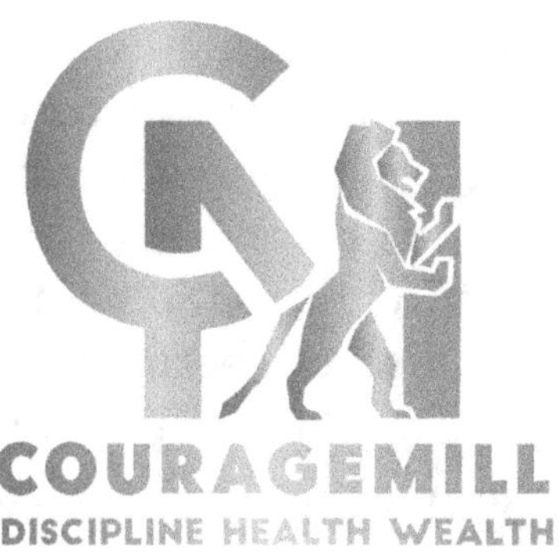

As I look back on my life, there was always some kind of addiction I was struggling with. I had my battles with drugs, alcohol, video games, TV shows and many more I couldn't recall. I never could have guessed that one addiction would have a profound impact on my health and well-being like my addiction to food. I was always taught that snaking was important to keep up energy levels. I was told that a great day started with a carbohydrate rich breakfast. Three plus meals a day was the pathway to good health. If I only knew then what I know now.

By the age of 28, I was diagnosed with cancer,

which metastasized with a 20% survival chance. I beat that cancer, but soon I would battle more cancer and other very serious health conditions. Most recently I was diagnosed with prediabetes, high blood pressure, high cholesterol, fatty liver, chronic kidney disease, peripheral neuropathy, sleep apnea, and I was 100 pounds overweight.

My doctor at the time had me on 9 different medications that only managed my symptoms. There was no cure apparently. I would live a short life, but I could be relatively symptom free while on these medications. Quality of life and lifespan reduced. I struggled with the prognosis and immediately began my search for a cure.

I refused to accept this, just as when I was diagnosed with severe cancer, rather than succumb, I decided to fight. During my search for a solution to my health woes, I came across some very compelling literature that associated overeating, sugar and carbohydrate consumption to all the metabolic syndrome x diseases I was battling with.

I continued to delve into this extremely controversial topic of the KETO diet and fasting as an alternative to prescription drugs. What I found was a cure and a lifestyle that has changed my life forever. After three years of intermittent and extended fasting, a sugar free and extremely reduced carbohydrate diet, I was able to cure everything, including severe peripheral neuropathy.

I am sure every person reading this book has experienced that deep tummy hunger grumble. Instantly you think "I'm Hungry". All these years I have been eating 3 meals a day plus snacks and drinks. How could I have known all these years. In an instant I realized I was the problem. I was caught in the Carb Trap and addicted. I feel obligated to share my story and outcome.

What I am about to share with you, is a culmination of everything that I have learned which saved my life, and even reversed my metabolic age. This information is invaluable and should be shared with the world. The pushback from mainstream medical and industrial pharmaceutical complex is staggering. I am not a doctor or an expert on diet health. I would however tell you to do your own research. Everyone may not have the same experience. Without any more delay let's delve into this book "Fasting Forward: A Journey Away from Addiction to Food."

UNDERSTANDING GLOBAL OBESITY RATES:

Causes, Consequences, and Solutions

"So we fasted and petitioned our God about this, and he answered our prayer." - Ezra 8:23 (NIV)

◆ ◆ ◆

Obesity has emerged as a global health epidemic, affecting individuals, communities, and economies worldwide. Over the past few decades, obesity rates have risen steadily across the globe, posing significant challenges to public health systems and societies at large. This first chapter explores the factors contributing to the rise in global obesity rates, its consequences on health and well-being, and potential strategies to address this pressing issue.

The Global Obesity Epidemic:

Obesity is defined as an excessive accumulation of body fat that poses health risks. The World Health Organization (WHO) recognizes obesity as a complex, multifactorial condition influenced by genetic, environmental, and behavioral factors. According to WHO, obesity has nearly tripled since 1975, with over 650 million adults and 340 million children classified as obese in 2016.

Factors Contributing to Obesity:

1. Dietary Patterns: The shift towards diets high in carbohydrates, calories, sugars, and processed foods has contributed significantly to rising obesity rates. The proliferation of fast-food chains, coupled with sedentary lifestyles, has led to increased consumption of energy-dense foods and decreased physical activity.

2. Sedentary Lifestyle: Technological advancements, urbanization, and changing work patterns have resulted in a decrease in physical activity levels. Sedentary behaviors such as prolonged screen time, commuting by car, and desk-bound jobs have become the norm in many societies, exacerbating the obesity epidemic.

3. Socioeconomic Factors: Obesity disproportionately affects populations with lower socioeconomic status due to limited access

to nutritious foods, opportunities for physical activity, and healthcare services. Socioeconomic disparities also contribute to higher rates of obesity-related comorbidities such as diabetes, cardiovascular diseases, and certain cancers, which studies show insulin resistance and diabetes have a significant effect on the development of these diseases.

4. Environmental Factors: Built environments that discourage walking or cycling, lack of safe recreational spaces, and advertising promoting unhealthy foods all contribute to the obesogenic environment. Additionally, food deserts—areas with limited access to affordable, nutritious foods —exacerbate the problem, particularly in urban areas.

5. Genetic and Biological Factors: While genetic predisposition plays a role in individual susceptibility to obesity, its rapid global spread suggests that environmental and behavioral factors are primary drivers of the epidemic. However, genetic factors may interact with environmental influences to exacerbate obesity risk in certain populations.

Obesity is associated with a myriad of health consequences, including:

1. Chronic Diseases: Obesity increases the risk of developing chronic conditions such as type 2 diabetes, hypertension, dyslipidemia,

cardiovascular diseases, stroke, and certain types of cancer. These conditions contribute to reduced quality of life, disability, and premature mortality.

2. Mental Health: Obesity is linked to psychological distress, low self-esteem, depression, and body image dissatisfaction, particularly among adolescents and young adults. Stigma and discrimination against individuals with obesity further exacerbate these mental health challenges.

3. Economic Burden: The economic costs of obesity are substantial, encompassing direct healthcare expenditures, productivity losses, absenteeism, and disability. Healthcare systems face increased financial strain due to the management of obesity-related conditions and complications.

4. Social Implications: Obesity can lead to social isolation, discrimination, and reduced opportunities in education, employment, and social participation. Weight bias and stigma perpetuate inequalities and hinder efforts to address the root causes of obesity.

Addressing the Obesity Epidemic:

Addressing the global obesity epidemic requires a multifaceted approach involving various stakeholders, including governments, healthcare systems, communities, and individuals. Key strategies include:

1. Promoting Healthy Diets: Implementing policies to improve food environments, such as taxation on sugary beverages, subsidies for fruits and vegetables, and food labeling initiatives, can encourage healthier dietary choices. Nutrition education and cooking skills programs also empower individuals to make informed decisions about their diets.

2. Encouraging Physical Activity: Creating walkable communities, investing in public transportation, and providing access to safe parks, playgrounds, and recreational facilities promote physical activity. Workplace wellness programs, school-based initiatives, and community fitness programs encourage regular exercise and active lifestyles.

3. Policy Interventions: Governments play a crucial role in implementing policies to address the structural determinants of obesity, including urban planning, transportation policies, agricultural subsidies, and food marketing regulations. Fiscal policies such as taxes on unhealthy foods and incentives for health-promoting behaviors can help shift societal norms towards healthier choices.

4. Healthcare Interventions: Healthcare systems should prioritize obesity prevention, early detection, and comprehensive management

through integrated care models. This includes screening for obesity-related comorbidities, providing access to evidence-based treatments, and promoting multidisciplinary approaches involving dieticians, psychologists, and exercise specialists.

5. Community Engagement: Engaging communities in grassroots initiatives, social marketing campaigns, and advocacy efforts fosters collective action and social support for obesity prevention. Empowering individuals and communities to create supportive environments for healthy living is essential for long-term success.

The global obesity epidemic represents one of the most significant public health challenges of the 21st century, with far-reaching consequences for individuals, communities, and societies. Addressing obesity requires a comprehensive, multisectoral approach that addresses its complex underlying determinants and promotes health equity. By implementing evidence-based strategies at the policy, environmental, and individual levels, we can mitigate the impact of obesity and create healthier, more sustainable futures for all.

While the concept of food addiction is not explicitly mentioned in the Bible, there are verses that touch upon the themes of self-control, moderation, and dependence. Here are five biblical quotes that relate to the concept of food addiction indirectly:

1. "Do not be with heavy drinkers of wine, Or with gluttonous eaters of meat; For the heavy drinker and the glutton will come to poverty, And drowsiness will clothe one with rags." - Proverbs 23:20-21 (NASB)

2. "All things are lawful for me, but not all things are profitable. All things are lawful for me, but I will not be mastered by anything." - 1 Corinthians 6:12 (NASB)

3. "So, whether you eat or drink, or whatever you do, do all to the glory of God." - 1 Corinthians 10:31 (ESV)

4. "For the desires of the flesh are against the Spirit, and the desires of the Spirit are against the flesh, for these are opposed to each other, to keep you from doing the things you want to do." - Galatians 5:17 (ESV)

5. "For we ourselves were once foolish, disobedient, led astray, slaves to various passions and pleasures, passing our days in malice and envy, hated by others and hating one another." - Titus 3:3 (ESV)

While these verses may not directly address food addiction, they highlight principles of self-control, moderation, and spiritual guidance that can be applied to overcoming unhealthy behaviors, including those related to food consumption.

CARBOHYDRATES AND HUNGER:

A Complex Relationship

"Food can be the most addictive substance in our lives, yet it's the one we need to survive."

◆ ◆ ◆

Carbohydrates, found abundantly in foods like grains, fruits, vegetables, and processed snacks, have long been associated with feelings of hunger and satiety. The intricate interplay between carbohydrates and hunger involves various physiological, hormonal, and psychological factors that influence appetite regulation and food intake. This chapter explores the multifaceted relationship between carbohydrates and hunger, examining the mechanisms behind carbohydrate-induced hunger, the impact of different types of carbohydrates on appetite, and practical strategies for managing hunger while optimizing dietary choices.

Understanding Carbohydrates and Hunger:

1. Carbohydrates and Energy:

- Energy Source: Carbohydrates are the body's primary source of energy, providing glucose, the simplest form of carbohydrate, for cellular metabolism and fueling metabolic processes. Glucose derived from dietary carbohydrates is readily absorbed into the bloodstream, where it serves as a readily available source of energy for tissues and organs.

- Blood Sugar Regulation: Carbohydrates influence blood sugar levels, which play a crucial role in appetite regulation and hunger signaling. High-carbohydrate meals can lead to rapid spikes in blood sugar followed by subsequent drops, triggering feelings of hunger and prompting further food consumption to maintain energy balance.

2. Hormonal Regulation:

- Insulin Response: Carbohydrate consumption stimulates the release of insulin, a hormone secreted by the pancreas in response to elevated blood glucose levels. Insulin facilitates the uptake of glucose into cells for energy production and storage, promoting glycogen synthesis in the liver and muscle tissue.

- Ghrelin and Leptin: Carbohydrates also influence hunger and satiety hormones, such as ghrelin and leptin, which regulate appetite and energy balance. Ghrelin, known as the hunger hormone, increases appetite and promotes food intake, while leptin, the satiety hormone, signals fullness and reduces hunger cues.

Mechanisms Behind Carbohydrate-Induced Hunger:

1. Blood Sugar Fluctuations:

- Glycemic Response: High-glycemic carbohydrates, such as refined grains, sugars, and processed foods, are rapidly digested and absorbed, leading to sharp increases in blood sugar levels followed by rapid declines. These fluctuations in blood sugar can trigger hunger pangs, cravings, and feelings of low energy, prompting individuals to seek out additional sources of carbohydrates to replenish energy stores.

- Hypoglycemia: Prolonged consumption of high-glycemic carbohydrates can contribute to reactive hypoglycemia, a condition characterized by low blood sugar levels following a meal. Hypoglycemia triggers hunger and cravings for sugary or carbohydrate-rich foods as the body seeks to restore blood glucose levels and alleviate symptoms of low energy and fatigue.

2. Insulin Resistance and Hunger:

- Insulin Dysregulation: Chronic consumption of high-carbohydrate diets can lead to insulin resistance, a condition in which cells become less responsive to insulin signaling, resulting in elevated blood sugar levels and compensatory increases in insulin secretion. Insulin resistance disrupts hunger and satiety signaling, leading to impaired appetite regulation and persistent feelings of hunger despite adequate energy intake.

- Hyperinsulinemia: Excessive insulin secretion in response to carbohydrate consumption can promote hunger and overeating by suppressing leptin signaling, increasing ghrelin production, and stimulating appetite centers in the brain. Hyperinsulinemia exacerbates carbohydrate cravings and reinforces the cycle of carbohydrate-induced hunger and overconsumption.

3. Neurotransmitter Imbalance:

- Dopamine and Serotonin: Carbohydrates influence neurotransmitter activity in the brain, particularly dopamine and serotonin, which play key roles in reward processing, mood regulation, and appetite control. Consumption of carbohydrate-rich foods can trigger the release of dopamine, the "feel-good" neurotransmitter, leading to temporary feelings of pleasure and satisfaction.

- Cravings and Emotional Eating: Carbohydrates, especially those high in sugar and refined grains, can promote cravings and emotional eating behaviors by modulating neurotransmitter activity and reinforcing reward pathways in the brain. Emotional triggers, stress, and environmental cues can exacerbate carbohydrate cravings and drive compulsive eating behaviors, independent of physiological hunger cues.

Impact of Different Types of Carbohydrates on Hunger:

1. Simple vs. Complex Carbohydrates:

- Simple Carbohydrates: Simple carbohydrates, such as sugars and refined grains, are quickly digested and absorbed, leading to rapid spikes in blood sugar followed by subsequent drops. Foods high in simple carbohydrates, such as candy, soda, and white bread, can promote hunger and cravings due to their high glycemic index and minimal satiating effect.

- Complex Carbohydrates: Complex carbohydrates, like such as leafy greens, mushrooms and other organic vegetables, are rich in fiber, vitamins, and minerals, and are digested more slowly, leading to gradual increases in blood sugar and sustained energy release. Consuming complex carbohydrates can promote satiety, stabilize blood sugar levels, and reduce feelings of hunger and overeating.

SNACKING:

Its Impact on Health and Well-being

Snacking has become a prevalent eating behavior in modern society, with many individuals consuming snacks between meals to satisfy hunger, boost energy, or simply indulge in flavorful treats. While snacking can offer convenience and enjoyment, it also raises concerns about its potential negative health effects. This chapter examines the relationship between snacking and health, exploring the physiological, psychological, and behavioral factors that contribute to the detrimental impact of excessive snacking on overall well-being.

Understanding Snacking Behavior:

1. Definition and Patterns of Snacking:

   - Snacking refers to the consumption of food

or beverages between regular meals, typically characterized by smaller portion sizes and a wide range of options, including both nutritious and indulgent choices. Snacking behaviors vary among individuals and cultures, influenced by factors such as dietary preferences, lifestyle habits, social norms, and environmental cues.

- Snacking Patterns: Snacking can occur at any time of the day, with common snacking occasions including mid-morning snacks, afternoon snacks, evening snacks, and late-night snacks. Snack choices may range from healthier options such as fruits, vegetables, nuts, and yogurt to less nutritious choices such as chips, cookies, candies, and sugary beverages.

2. Factors Influencing Snacking Behavior:

- Hunger and Appetite: Snacking is often driven by feelings of hunger, appetite, or cravings between meals, as individuals seek to alleviate physical sensations of hunger or satisfy taste preferences. Appetite cues, environmental triggers, emotional states, and social influences can all contribute to the decision to snack, regardless of actual energy needs.

- Emotional Eating: Emotional factors, such as stress, boredom, sadness, or loneliness, can prompt individuals to turn to food for comfort, distraction, or emotional regulation. Emotional eating behaviors may lead to mindless snacking, excessive calorie intake, and negative feelings of guilt or remorse afterward.

- Social and Environmental Cues: Social settings, cultural norms, advertising, and food availability in the environment can influence snacking behaviors by promoting certain foods, creating opportunities for grazing, or encouraging social eating occasions. Peer pressure, social gatherings, and workplace environments may also influence snacking choices and frequency.

Negative Health Effects of Excessive Snacking:

1. Weight Gain and Obesity:

- Excess Caloric Intake: Frequent snacking, especially on high-calorie, nutrient-poor foods, can contribute to an overall increase in daily calorie consumption, leading to weight gain and obesity over time. Snacking between meals adds extra calories to the diet, often without providing essential nutrients or promoting satiety, which can disrupt energy balance and contribute to positive energy balance.

- Energy Imbalance: Continuous grazing or frequent snacking throughout the day may disrupt the body's natural hunger and satiety cues, leading to overeating and a chronic surplus of energy intake. This imbalance between energy intake and expenditure can promote fat storage, adiposity, and weight gain, increasing the risk of obesity-related health complications such as type 2 diabetes, cardiovascular disease, and metabolic syndrome.

2. Poor Nutrient Intake:

- Nutrient Dilution: Excessive snacking on processed, energy-dense foods may displace nutrient-rich foods from the diet, leading to inadequate intake of essential vitamins, minerals, fiber, and phytonutrients. Snack foods high in added sugars, refined grains, unhealthy fats, and sodium provide empty calories and minimal nutritional value, contributing to nutrient dilution and suboptimal dietary quality.

- Micronutrient Deficiencies: Regular consumption of snack foods low in essential nutrients, such as fruits, vegetables, whole grains, and lean proteins, can increase the risk of micronutrient deficiencies and nutrient imbalances. Inadequate intake of vitamins, minerals, and antioxidants may compromise immune function, bone health, cognitive function, and overall well-being, exacerbating the negative health effects of excessive snacking.

3. Disrupted Blood Sugar Regulation:

- Blood Sugar Spikes and Crashes: Snacking on high-carbohydrate, high-glycemic foods can lead to rapid spikes in blood sugar levels followed by subsequent crashes, triggering fluctuations in energy, mood, and appetite. The consumption of sugary snacks, refined carbohydrates, and sweetened beverages can disrupt blood sugar regulation, leading to insulin resistance, metabolic dysfunction, and increased risk of type 2 diabetes.

- Insulin Resistance: Chronic snacking on carbohydrate-rich foods can contribute to insulin resistance, a condition in which cells become less responsive to insulin signaling, leading to elevated blood sugar levels and compensatory increases in insulin secretion. Insulin resistance disrupts glucose metabolism, promotes fat storage, and increases the risk of metabolic disorders associated with dysregulated blood sugar control.

4. Dental Health Issues:

- Dental Erosion and Decay: Snacking on sugary, acidic, or sticky foods can increase the risk of dental erosion, enamel erosion, and tooth decay. Frequent exposure to sugary snacks, candies, sodas, and sweetened beverages can create an acidic environment in the mouth, leading to demineralization of tooth enamel, cavity formation, and dental caries. Snacking habits that involve prolonged consumption of snacks or beverages with high sugar content, especially without proper oral hygiene practices, can accelerate tooth decay and compromise oral health.

5. Digestive Discomfort and Gut Health:

- Digestive Issues: Excessive snacking, particularly on foods high in refined carbohydrates, added sugars, and unhealthy fats, can disrupt digestive function and lead to symptoms such as bloating, gas, indigestion, and gastrointestinal discomfort. Snack foods low in fiber and nutrients may lack the dietary components needed to support optimal digestion and gut health.

- Microbiome Imbalance: Imbalanced snacking patterns may negatively impact the gut microbiota, the community of microorganisms residing in the gastrointestinal tract that play a crucial role in digestion, nutrient absorption, immune function, and metabolic health. Consuming a diet high in processed snacks and low in fiber-rich foods can alter the composition and diversity of gut bacteria, increasing the risk of dysbiosis, inflammation, and gastrointestinal disorders.

6. Psychological Effects and Food Relationships:

- Emotional Eating Patterns: Excessive snacking can contribute to maladaptive eating behaviors, such as emotional eating, stress eating, and binge eating, which are driven by psychological factors rather than physiological hunger cues. Using snacks as a coping mechanism for stress, boredom, or negative emotions can create an unhealthy relationship with food, leading to disordered eating patterns and negative psychological outcomes.

- Guilt and Shame: Feelings of guilt, shame, or self-judgment often accompany episodes of overeating or indulging in unhealthy snacks, particularly when snacking occurs in response to emotional triggers or cravings. Negative emotions associated with food choices can perpetuate a cycle of emotional eating, restrict-binge cycles, and contribute to poor self-esteem, body dissatisfaction, and mental health issues.

Practical Strategies for Promoting Healthy Snacking Habits:

While healthy snacking habits can help those that struggle with discipline, I would argue that snacking in general is unhealthy because of the continuous release of insulin which can lead to insulin resistance. Here are some helpful tips on healthy snacking habits.

1. Choose Nutrient-Dense Snacks:

- Whole Foods: Opt for whole, minimally processed snacks that provide essential nutrients, vitamins, minerals, and dietary fiber to support overall health and well-being. Choose nutrient-dense options such as fruits, vegetables, nuts, seeds, whole grains, and dairy products without added sugars or unhealthy additives.

- Balanced Macronutrients: Incorporate snacks that contain a balance of carbohydrates, proteins, and healthy fats to promote satiety, stabilize blood sugar levels, and sustain energy throughout the day. Pairing carbohydrates with protein or fiber-rich foods can help mitigate blood sugar spikes and enhance feelings of fullness and satisfaction.

2. Practice Portion Control:

- Mindful Portions: Practice portion control when snacking by measuring serving sizes, using small plates or bowls, and avoiding mindless eating in front of screens or while distracted. Pay attention to hunger and satiety cues and stop eating when you feel comfortably satisfied rather than overly full.

- Pre-portioned Snacks: Pre-portioned snacks into single-serving containers or bags to avoid overeating and promote mindful consumption. Preparing snacks ahead of time can help prevent impulsive snacking and encourage healthier choices throughout the day.

3. Emphasize Whole, Plant-Based Foods:

- Fruits and Vegetables: Increase consumption of fruits and vegetables as convenient, nutrient-rich snack options that provide vitamins, minerals, antioxidants, and dietary fiber. Fresh, frozen, or dried fruits and vegetables can satisfy sweet or savory cravings while supporting overall health and hydration.

- Plant-Based Proteins: Include plant-based protein sources such as nuts, seeds, legumes, tofu, and edamame as satiating snacks that provide essential amino acids, healthy fats, and micronutrients. Plant-based proteins offer a sustainable and environmentally friendly alternative to animal-derived snacks.

4. Mindful Eating Practices:

- Conscious Snacking: Practice mindful eating techniques, such as eating slowly, savoring each bite, and paying attention to taste, texture, and satiety signals. Mindful snacking encourages greater awareness of food choices, portion sizes, and eating behaviors, fostering a positive relationship with food and promoting mindful consumption.

- Emotional Awareness: Recognize emotional triggers, stressors, or environmental cues that may prompt snacking behaviors and seek alternative coping strategies or distractions to address emotional hunger. Engage in stress-reduction techniques, such as deep breathing, meditation, or physical activity, to manage emotions and reduce reliance on food for comfort.

5. Hydration and Beverage Choices:

- Water Intake: Stay hydrated throughout the day by drinking water between meals to support hydration, promote satiety, and prevent dehydration-related hunger cues. Opt for water as the primary beverage choice, and limit consumption of sugary drinks, sweetened beverages, and caffeinated products that can contribute to excess calorie intake and disrupt hydration balance.

- Herbal Teas: Enjoy herbal teas or infusions as calorie-free alternatives to sugary snacks or beverages, providing hydration, flavor, and relaxation without added sugars or artificial additives. Herbal teas can satisfy cravings for warmth, sweetness, or flavor while promoting feelings of calmness and well-being.

While snacking can offer convenience, pleasure, and occasional indulgence, excessive snacking and poor snack choices can have negative implications for overall health and well-being. The detrimental effects of frequent snacking extend beyond weight gain and obesity to encompass poor nutrient intake, disrupted blood sugar regulation, dental health issues, digestive discomfort, psychological distress, and disordered eating patterns. However, with mindful awareness and strategic planning, individuals can adopt healthier snacking habits and mitigate the adverse consequences associated with excessive snacking.

By choosing nutrient-dense snacks, practicing portion control, emphasizing whole, plant-based foods, incorporating mindful eating practices, and prioritizing hydration and beverage choices, individuals can promote satiety, stabilize blood sugar levels, and support overall health while enjoying satisfying snack options. Additionally, addressing emotional triggers, stressors, and environmental cues that contribute to snacking behaviors can help individuals develop a healthier relationship with food and cultivate mindfulness in eating habits.

Education, awareness, and access to nutritious snack options are essential components of promoting healthy snacking habits and empowering individuals to make informed dietary choices. Healthcare professionals, educators, and policymakers play a crucial role in disseminating evidence-based information, promoting nutritional literacy, and creating environments conducive to healthy eating behaviors. By fostering a culture of mindful eating, moderation, and self-awareness, we can empower individuals to navigate the complex landscape of snacking while prioritizing their health and well-being.

In conclusion, snacking can either contribute to or detract from overall health and well-being, depending on the choices we make and the habits we cultivate. By adopting a balanced approach to snacking, incorporating nutrient-rich foods, and practicing mindful eating, individuals can enjoy the benefits of snacking while minimizing the potential negative health effects. Through education, awareness, and conscious decision-making, we can harness the power of snacking to nourish our bodies, support our health goals, and enhance our quality of life.

THE CORRELATION:

Diabetes and Heart Disease, Cancer, and Other Metabolic Diseases

"Do not be with heavy drinkers of wine, Or with gluttonous eaters of meat; For the heavy drinker and the glutton will come to poverty, And drowsiness will clothe one with rags." - Proverbs 23:20-21 (NASB)

◆ ◆ ◆

Diabetes mellitus, a metabolic disorder characterized by elevated blood glucose levels, is a significant public health concern worldwide. Beyond its immediate health implications, diabetes is associated with an increased risk of developing various comorbidities, including heart disease, cancer, and other metabolic disorders. This chapter delves into the intricate relationship between diabetes and these conditions, highlighting the underlying mechanisms, epidemiological evidence, and clinical implications.

Diabetes and Heart Disease:

1. Epidemiological Evidence:

-    Individuals with diabetes are at a substantially higher risk of developing cardiovascular diseases (CVD), including coronary artery disease, stroke, and peripheral vascular disease.

-    According to the American Heart Association, adults with diabetes are two to four times more likely to die from heart disease than those without diabetes.

- Diabetes accelerates the progression of atherosclerosis, the underlying cause of most CVD, through mechanisms involving chronic inflammation, endothelial dysfunction, and dyslipidemia.

- Poorly controlled diabetes exacerbates traditional CVD risk factors such as hypertension, dyslipidemia, and obesity, further increasing the risk of cardiovascular events.

2. Underlying Mechanisms:

- Hyperglycemia: Prolonged exposure to high

blood glucose levels promotes oxidative stress, inflammation, and endothelial dysfunction, contributing to the development and progression of atherosclerosis.

- Insulin Resistance: Insulin resistance, a hallmark of type 2 diabetes, is associated with dyslipidemia, hypertension, and central obesity —key components of the metabolic syndrome, which predisposes individuals to CVD.

- Dyslipidemia: Diabetes alters lipid metabolism, leading to elevated levels of triglycerides, low-density lipoprotein cholesterol, and decreased levels of high-density lipoprotein cholesterol, all of which contribute to atherosclerosis.

- Inflammatory Pathways: Diabetes induces a chronic inflammatory state characterized by increased levels of pro-inflammatory cytokines, adhesion molecules, and acute-phase reactants, further promoting atherosclerosis and vascular damage.

Diabetes and Cancer:

1. Epidemiological Evidence:

- Epidemiological studies have consistently demonstrated an association between diabetes and an increased risk of various cancers, including pancreatic, liver, colorectal, breast, and bladder cancer.

- The link between diabetes and cancer is bidirectional, with diabetes increasing the risk of certain cancers, while some cancers may predispose individuals to diabetes due to cancer-related metabolic alterations and treatments.

- Obesity, insulin resistance, hyperinsulinemia, chronic inflammation, and dysregulated growth factor signaling pathways contribute to the pathophysiological links between diabetes and cancer.

2. Underlying Mechanisms:

- Hyperinsulinemia: Insulin exerts mitogenic effects on cells, promoting cell proliferation, survival, and tumor growth. Chronic hyperinsulinemia, a hallmark of insulin resistance and type 2 diabetes, stimulates insulin-like growth factor-1 (IGF-1) signaling, which plays a key role in cancer development and progression.

- Dysregulated Growth Factors: Insulin and IGF-1 signaling pathways promote tumorigenesis by activating oncogenic pathways, inhibiting apoptosis, and enhancing angiogenesis and metastasis.

- Chronic Inflammation: Diabetes-induced inflammation contributes to cancer development through the production of pro-inflammatory cytokines, chemokines, and reactive oxygen species, which promote genomic instability and oncogenic mutations.

- Shared Risk Factors: Obesity, physical inactivity, unhealthy dietary patterns, and smoking—common risk factors for both diabetes and cancer—further contribute to the observed association between the two conditions.

Diabetes and Other Metabolic Diseases:

1. Non-Alcoholic Fatty Liver Disease (NAFLD):

- NAFLD, characterized by excessive hepatic fat accumulation in the absence of significant alcohol consumption, is strongly associated with insulin resistance, obesity, and type 2 diabetes.

- Insulin resistance and dyslipidemia contribute to hepatic lipid accumulation, inflammation, and oxidative stress, leading to the progression of NAFLD to non-alcoholic steatohepatitis (NASH) and eventually liver fibrosis, cirrhosis, and hepatocellular carcinoma.

- Management of diabetes focuses on optimizing glycemic control, weight loss, and lifestyle modifications to mitigate the risk of NAFLD progression and associated complications.

2. Chronic Kidney Disease (CKD):

- Diabetes is the leading cause of CKD worldwide, accounting for approximately one-third of all cases of end-stage renal disease (ESRD).

- Hyperglycemia, hypertension, dyslipidemia, and systemic inflammation contribute to the development and progression of diabetic nephropathy, a major complication of diabetes characterized by glomerular injury, proteinuria, and declining renal function.

- Tight glycemic and blood pressure control, renin-angiotensin-aldosterone system blockade, and lifestyle interventions are essential in preventing and managing diabetic kidney disease.

The correlation between diabetes and heart disease, cancer, and other metabolic diseases underscores the importance of comprehensive management strategies that address the underlying pathophysiological mechanisms and shared risk factors.

Early detection, aggressive risk factor modification, lifestyle interventions, and multidisciplinary care are paramount in reducing the burden of diabetes-related comorbidities and improving overall health outcomes.

A holistic approach that integrates preventive measures, patient education, and evidence-based therapies is essential in mitigating the adverse effects of diabetes on cardiovascular, oncological, and metabolic health.

GUT HEALTH:

Understanding the Negative Effects and Implications

❖ ❖ ❖

Gut microbiota, comprising trillions of microorganisms residing in the gastrointestinal tract, plays a crucial role in maintaining digestive health, immune function, and metabolic homeostasis. Emerging research has shed light on the detrimental effects of excessive sugar and carbohydrate consumption on gut microbiota composition, intestinal barrier integrity, and inflammatory responses, with implications for overall health and well-being. This chapter delves into the negative impact of sugar and carbohydrates on gut health, elucidating the underlying mechanisms, clinical manifestations, and therapeutic strategies for mitigating their adverse effects.

Understanding Gut Health:

1. Gut Microbiota:

- Microbial Diversity: The gut harbors a diverse ecosystem of bacteria, fungi, viruses, and archaea, collectively known as the gut microbiota. Microbial diversity and composition vary among individuals and are influenced by factors such as diet, lifestyle, genetics, and environmental exposures.

- Microbiota Functions: The gut microbiota performs vital functions, including fermentation of dietary fibers, production of short-chain fatty acids (SCFAs), synthesis of vitamins and neurotransmitters, and modulation of immune responses. A balanced microbiota contributes to gastrointestinal homeostasis, mucosal integrity, and host-microbe symbiosis.

2. Intestinal Barrier:

- Intestinal Epithelium: The intestinal epithelium serves as a physical barrier between the gut lumen and underlying tissues, preventing the translocation of harmful microorganisms, toxins, and antigens into systemic circulation. Tight junction proteins, such as occludin and claudins, regulate paracellular permeability and maintain barrier function.

- Mucus Layer: The mucus layer, produced by

goblet cells, forms an additional protective barrier in the gut, shielding the epithelium from luminal contents and facilitating microbial colonization. Disruption of the mucus layer compromises barrier integrity and predisposes to microbial invasion and inflammation.

Negative Effects of Sugar and Carbohydrates on Gut Health:

1. Dysbiosis:

- Altered Microbial Composition: High-sugar diets and refined carbohydrate intake promote dysbiosis—a disruption of the gut microbiota characterized by shifts in microbial diversity and abundance. Excessive sugar consumption favors the growth of pro-inflammatory bacteria (e.g., Firmicutes) and reduces beneficial bacteria (e.g., Bacteroidetes), leading to microbial imbalances associated with gastrointestinal disorders.

- Reduction in Beneficial Species: Sugars and refined carbohydrates provide substrates for pathogenic bacteria, such as Clostridium difficile and Enterobacteriaceae, while depleting populations of beneficial commensals, such as Bifidobacteria and Lactobacilli. Dysbiosis alters microbial metabolite production, impairs SCFA synthesis, and disrupts host-microbe interactions critical for gut homeostasis.

- Increased Pathogen Susceptibility: Dysbiotic

changes in the gut microbiota compromise colonization resistance, allowing opportunistic pathogens to proliferate and cause infections. Disrupted microbial ecosystems promote overgrowth of pathogenic species, colonization of mucosal surfaces, and invasion of epithelial tissues, leading to acute and chronic gastrointestinal infections.

2. Intestinal Inflammation:

- Immune Dysregulation: Sugar-induced dysbiosis and alterations in gut microbiota composition trigger immune dysregulation, characterized by aberrant immune activation, cytokine production, and inflammatory responses in the intestinal mucosa. Chronic low-grade inflammation contributes to mucosal injury, barrier dysfunction, and perpetuation of inflammatory cascades implicated in gastrointestinal diseases.

- Endotoxemia: Dysbiotic changes in the gut microbiota promote the release of bacterial lipopolysaccharides (LPS) and other microbial products into systemic circulation, triggering systemic inflammation and metabolic disturbances. Endotoxemia, resulting from increased intestinal permeability and translocation of microbial toxins, exacerbates insulin resistance, oxidative stress, and inflammatory conditions associated with metabolic syndrome.

- Gut-Brain Axis Dysfunction: Intestinal inflammation and dysbiosis disrupt communication along the gut-brain axis—a bidirectional signaling pathway linking the gut microbiota, enteric nervous system, and central nervous system. Dysfunctional gut-brain axis signaling contributes to mood disorders, cognitive impairment, and psychiatric symptoms observed in individuals with gastrointestinal disorders and inflammatory bowel diseases.

3. Impaired Gut Barrier Function:

- Increased Permeability: Sugar consumption and refined carbohydrate intake compromise intestinal barrier function by disrupting tight junction integrity, reducing mucin production, and promoting epithelial damage. Increased gut permeability, or "leaky gut," allows the translocation of luminal antigens, endotoxins, and microbial metabolites across the epithelial barrier, triggering immune responses and systemic inflammation.

- Mucosal Damage: Sugar-induced inflammation and oxidative stress impair mucosal repair mechanisms, exacerbating epithelial injury and compromising barrier integrity. Disrupted epithelial tight junctions facilitate paracellular flux of macromolecules, pathogens, and inflammatory mediators, perpetuating mucosal damage and intestinal inflammation in gastrointestinal disorders.

Clinical Manifestations and Disease Associations:

1. Gastrointestinal Disorders:

   - Irritable Bowel Syndrome (IBS): Sugar-rich diets exacerbate symptoms of irritable bowel syndrome, including abdominal pain, bloating, diarrhea, and constipation, by inducing dysbiosis, mucosal inflammation, and visceral hypersensitivity. FODMAPs (fermentable oligosaccharides, disaccharides, monosaccharides, and polyols), a group of fermentable carbohydrates present in certain foods, trigger gastrointestinal symptoms in susceptible individuals with IBS.

   - Inflammatory Bowel Disease (IBD): Excessive sugar consumption is associated with an increased risk of inflammatory bowel diseases, such as Crohn's disease and ulcerative colitis, characterized by chronic intestinal inflammation and mucosal damage. Sugar-induced dysbiosis and immune dysregulation contribute to disease exacerbations, mucosal injury, and disease progression in individuals with IBD.

2. Metabolic Disorders:

- Obesity and Metabolic Syndrome: High-sugar diets contribute to obesity and metabolic syndrome by promoting insulin resistance, adipose tissue inflammation, and dyslipidemia. Sugar-induced dysbiosis alters energy harvest from the diet, enhances adipogenesis, and exacerbates systemic inflammation, predisposing individuals to obesity-related comorbidities, such as type 2 diabetes, cardiovascular diseases, and fatty liver disease.

- Non-Alcoholic Fatty Liver Disease (NAFLD): Excessive sugar consumption promotes hepatic lipogenesis, triglyceride accumulation, and insulin resistance in the liver, leading to non-alcoholic fatty liver disease—a spectrum of liver disorders ranging from simple steatosis to steatohepatitis and cirrhosis. Sugar-induced dysbiosis exacerbates hepatic inflammation, oxidative stress, and fibrosis progression in individuals with NAFLD.

3. Immune Disorders:

- Food Allergies and Intolerances: Sugar-rich diets and refined carbohydrate consumption contribute to the development of food allergies and intolerances by disrupting gut barrier function, altering mucosal immune responses, and modulating microbial interactions in the gut. Dysbiotic changes in the gut microbiota increase susceptibility to food sensitivities, allergic reactions, and autoimmune disorders characterized by dysregulated immune responses to dietary antigens.

- Celiac Disease: Sugars and refined carbohydrates exacerbate symptoms of celiac disease—a gluten-related autoimmune disorder characterized by intestinal inflammation, villous atrophy, and malabsorption of nutrients—in susceptible individuals with genetic predispositions. High-sugar diets promote dysbiosis, intestinal permeability, and immune activation, exacerbating gluten-induced mucosal damage and systemic inflammation in individuals with celiac disease.

4. Neurological and Psychiatric Disorders:

- Mood Disorders: Sugar consumption and refined carbohydrate intake influence mood and mental health outcomes by modulating neurotransmitter synthesis, gut-brain axis signaling, and inflammatory pathways implicated in mood regulation. Dysbiotic changes in the gut microbiota alter serotonin production, dopamine signaling, and GABAergic neurotransmission, contributing to mood disorders, such as depression, anxiety, and stress-related conditions.

- Neurodegenerative Diseases: Excessive sugar consumption exacerbates neuroinflammation, oxidative stress, and mitochondrial dysfunction in the brain, increasing the risk of neurodegenerative diseases, such as Alzheimer's disease, Parkinson's disease, and multiple sclerosis. Sugar-induced dysbiosis compromises the integrity of the blood-brain barrier, facilitates neurotoxin entry into the brain, and exacerbates neuronal damage and cognitive decline in neurodegenerative disorders.

Therapeutic Strategies for Promoting Gut Health:

1. Dietary Modifications:

- Low-Sugar Diet: Adopting a low-sugar diet, rich in fiber, phytonutrients, and prebiotic foods, supports gut health by reducing sugar-induced dysbiosis, inflammation, and intestinal permeability. Emphasizing whole foods, such as fruits, vegetables, legumes, and whole grains, provides essential nutrients, antioxidants, and dietary fibers that promote microbial diversity and fermentation in the gut.

- Mediterranean Diet: The Mediterranean diet, characterized by high consumption of plant-based foods, fish, olive oil, and moderate intake of red wine, offers protective benefits against gut-related diseases by promoting microbial balance, mucosal integrity, and anti-inflammatory responses. Mediterranean dietary patterns emphasize diversity, freshness, and seasonality of foods, aligning with principles of gut-friendly eating.

2. Probiotic and Prebiotic Supplementation:

-        Probiotics: Probiotic supplements containing beneficial bacterial strains, such as Lactobacillus and Bifidobacterium species, help restore microbial balance, enhance immune function, and alleviate gastrointestinal symptoms associated with sugar-induced dysbiosis. Probiotic supplementation may mitigate the adverse effects of high-sugar diets on gut health and promote microbial diversity in susceptible individuals.

- Prebiotics: Prebiotic fibers, such as inulin, oligofructose, and resistant starch, serve as substrates for beneficial bacteria in the gut, promoting their growth, fermentation, and production of SCFAs. Prebiotic supplementation enhances microbial diversity, mucosal barrier function, and metabolic health, mitigating the effects of sugar-induced dysbiosis and intestinal inflammation.

3. Lifestyle Modifications:

- Stress Management: Chronic stress disrupts gut-brain axis signaling, alters gut microbiota composition, and exacerbates gastrointestinal symptoms in susceptible individuals. Stress reduction techniques, such as mindfulness meditation, yoga, and relaxation therapies, promote psychological well-being, modulate neuroendocrine responses, and improve gut health outcomes.

- Physical Activity: Regular physical exercise enhances gut motility, microbial diversity, and intestinal barrier function, reducing the risk of gastrointestinal disorders and inflammatory conditions associated with sugar consumption. Aerobic exercise, resistance training, and outdoor activities support overall health and well-being by promoting metabolic health and immune function.

4. Medical Interventions:

- Gut Microbiota Modulation: Emerging therapeutic strategies, such as fecal microbiota transplantation (FMT), microbial-based therapies, and microbial metabolite supplementation, aim to restore gut microbiota balance, resilience, and functionality in individuals with dysbiosis-related disorders. Gut microbiota modulation holds promise for treating gastrointestinal diseases, metabolic disorders, and immune-mediated conditions by targeting microbial imbalances and dysregulated host-microbe interactions.

The negative effects of sugar and carbohydrates on gut health are multifaceted, encompassing dysbiosis, intestinal inflammation, impaired barrier function, and systemic repercussions affecting various organ systems.

By understanding the intricate interplay between dietary factors, gut microbiota composition, and host physiology, healthcare providers can implement targeted interventions aimed at promoting gut health, preventing disease progression, and optimizing overall well-being.

Embracing a holistic approach to gut health management, encompassing dietary modifications, lifestyle interventions, and medical therapies, empowers individuals to make informed choices that support gastrointestinal health and enhance resilience against the adverse effects of sugar and carbohydrates on the gut microbiome.

Through interdisciplinary collaboration, education, and research efforts, we can advance our understanding of gut-related diseases and develop innovative strategies for promoting gut health and improving quality of life for individuals worldwide.

INSULIN RESISTANCE:

*Early Onset Detection
Challenges*

◆ ◆ ◆

Insulin resistance, a metabolic condition characterized by impaired cellular response to insulin, represents a significant health concern with far-reaching implications for individuals and healthcare systems worldwide. Despite its insidious nature, insulin resistance often remains undetected in its early stages, posing challenges for timely intervention and prevention of associated complications. This chapter aims to elucidate the concept of insulin resistance, explore its early onset, and discuss the obstacles to its detection and management.

Understanding Insulin Resistance:

Insulin, a hormone produced by the pancreas, plays a crucial role in regulating glucose metabolism, lipid synthesis, and protein synthesis in target tissues such as liver, muscle, and adipose tissue. Insulin resistance occurs when these tissues become less responsive to the effects of insulin, leading to compensatory hyperinsulinemia and dysregulated glucose homeostasis. Over time, insulin resistance can progress to impaired glucose tolerance, prediabetes, and ultimately type 2 diabetes mellitus.

Early Onset of Insulin Resistance:

1. Predisposing Factors:

-       Genetic   Susceptibility: Genetic predisposition plays a significant role in the development of insulin resistance, with certain genetic variants affecting insulin signaling pathways, glucose transporters, and pancreatic beta-cell function.

- Lifestyle Factors: Sedentary behavior, excessive calorie intake, poor dietary choices (highly processed foods, sugary beverages), and obesity are major contributors to the early onset of insulin resistance. Excessive visceral adiposity, in particular, is strongly associated with insulin resistance and metabolic dysfunction.

- Gestational Factors: Intrauterine exposure to maternal obesity, gestational diabetes, and fetal overnutrition can predispose individuals to insulin resistance from early life, increasing the risk of metabolic disturbances in adulthood.

2. Childhood Insulin Resistance:

-      Childhood obesity rates have reached epidemic proportions globally, with approximately 38 million children under the age of 5 being overweight or obese.

- Pediatric obesity is strongly associated with insulin resistance, dyslipidemia, hypertension, and non-alcoholic fatty liver disease (NAFLD), collectively termed as metabolic syndrome in children.

- Insulin resistance in childhood sets the stage for the development of type 2 diabetes, cardiovascular diseases, and other metabolic disorders later in life, highlighting the importance of early intervention and prevention efforts.

Challenges in Early Detection of Insulin Resistance:

1. Lack of Symptomatic Presentation:

-      Insulin resistance often manifests asymptomatically in its early stages, making it challenging to detect clinically.

- While hyperinsulinemia and compensatory hyperglycemia may occur in response to insulin resistance, overt symptoms such as fatigue, polyuria, and polydipsia typically manifest only in advanced stages of glucose dysregulation.

- As a result, individuals with insulin resistance may remain undiagnosed until complications such as prediabetes, type 2 diabetes, or cardiovascular diseases emerge, highlighting the importance of proactive screening and risk assessment.

2. Diagnostic Limitations:

- Gold standard methods for assessing insulin sensitivity, such as the hyperinsulinemic-euglycemic clamp and the frequently sampled intravenous glucose tolerance test, are invasive, time-consuming, and impractical for routine clinical use.

- Surrogate markers of insulin resistance, including fasting insulin levels, homeostatic model assessment of insulin resistance (HOMA-IR), and quantitative insulin sensitivity check index (QUICKI), have limitations in terms of accuracy and reproducibility, particularly in heterogeneous populations.

3. Lack of Consensus on Screening Guidelines:

- Despite the growing prevalence of insulin resistance and its associated complications, there is a lack of consensus among healthcare organizations regarding screening guidelines for asymptomatic individuals.

- Screening recommendations vary based on age, sex, ethnicity, and presence of risk factors such as obesity, family history of diabetes, and history of gestational diabetes.

- In the absence of standardized screening protocols, many individuals at high risk for insulin resistance may go undetected, delaying the implementation of preventive measures and lifestyle interventions.

Management Strategies for Insulin Resistance:

1. Lifestyle Modifications:

- Lifestyle interventions focusing on diet, exercise, and weight management are cornerstone strategies for preventing and managing insulin resistance.

- A balanced diet rich in non-starchy vegetables, lean and fatty proteins, and healthy fats, coupled with regular physical activity, promotes weight loss, improves insulin sensitivity, and reduces the risk of metabolic complications.

- Behavioral interventions, nutrition counseling, and physical activity programs tailored to individual needs and preferences are essential components of comprehensive lifestyle modification plans.

2. Pharmacological Interventions:

- Pharmacotherapy may be considered in individuals with persistent insulin resistance despite lifestyle modifications or those at high risk for progression to diabetes or cardiovascular diseases.

- Insulin-sensitizing agents such as metformin, thiazolidinediones, and glucagon-like peptide-1 (GLP-1) receptor agonists are commonly used to improve insulin sensitivity, glycemic control, and metabolic parameters in patients with insulin resistance and prediabetes.

- Combination therapies targeting multiple metabolic pathways may be employed to achieve optimal outcomes and reduce the risk of long-term complications.

Insulin resistance represents a silent yet formidable threat to global health, predisposing individuals to a spectrum of metabolic disturbances and chronic diseases. Despite its early onset, insulin resistance often evades detection until complications arise, highlighting the urgent need for proactive screening, risk assessment, and intervention strategies. Addressing the challenges associated with early detection of insulin resistance requires a concerted effort from healthcare providers, policymakers, and communities to implement evidence-based screening protocols, promote lifestyle modifications, and facilitate access to comprehensive care. By recognizing the early signs of insulin resistance and intervening promptly, we can mitigate its adverse health consequences and improve the overall well-being of individuals at risk.

THE LINK AND CORRELATION:

Insulin Resistance, High Blood Pressure, and Arteriosclerosis

◆ ◆ ◆

Insulin resistance, a metabolic condition characterized by impaired cellular response to insulin, has garnered significant attention in the realm of cardiovascular health due to its association with hypertension and arteriosclerosis. The intricate interplay between insulin resistance, high blood pressure, and arteriosclerosis underscores the multifaceted nature of cardiovascular disease pathophysiology. This chapter aims to elucidate the underlying mechanisms linking insulin resistance to hypertension and arteriosclerosis, explore the epidemiological evidence supporting their correlation, and discuss the clinical implications of this association.

Insulin Resistance and Hypertension:

1. Underlying Mechanisms:

- Renal Sodium Retention: Insulin resistance disrupts renal sodium handling mechanisms, leading to increased sodium reabsorption in the proximal tubules and reduced sodium excretion. This results in expanded extracellular fluid volume, activation of the renin-angiotensin-aldosterone system (RAAS), and subsequent elevation of blood pressure.

- Endothelial Dysfunction: Insulin resistance is associated with impaired endothelial function, characterized by reduced nitric oxide bioavailability, increased endothelin-1 production, and enhanced vascular smooth muscle contraction. Endothelial dysfunction contributes to vasoconstriction, endothelial inflammation, and hypertension.

- Sympathetic Nervous System Activation: Insulin resistance is accompanied by sympathetic nervous system overactivity, characterized by increased sympathetic tone, elevated plasma catecholamine levels, and enhanced renal and vascular adrenergic responsiveness. Sympathetic activation contributes to increased vascular resistance, cardiac output, and blood pressure.

- Hyperinsulinemia and Insulin Signaling:

Chronic hyperinsulinemia, a compensatory response to insulin resistance, promotes sodium retention, sympathetic activation, and vascular smooth muscle proliferation through insulin-mediated signaling pathways. Dysregulated insulin signaling exacerbates hypertension by disrupting the balance between vasodilatory and vasoconstrictive pathways.

2. Epidemiological Evidence:

- Numerous epidemiological studies have demonstrated a strong association between insulin resistance and hypertension, independent of traditional cardiovascular risk factors.

- The Framingham Heart Study and other large-scale cohorts have reported that individuals with insulin resistance or hyperinsulinemia are at increased risk of developing hypertension over time, even after adjusting for confounding variables.

- Longitudinal studies have shown that insulin resistance precedes the onset of hypertension in a substantial proportion of cases, highlighting its role as a precursor to cardiovascular disease.

Insulin Resistance and Arteriosclerosis:

1. Atherosclerosis Pathogenesis:

- Insulin resistance contributes to the pathogenesis of arteriosclerosis, particularly atherosclerosis, through multiple mechanisms involving endothelial dysfunction, dyslipidemia, inflammation, and oxidative stress.

- Endothelial Dysfunction: Insulin resistance impairs endothelial function by reducing nitric oxide bioavailability, promoting endothelial activation, and increasing vascular permeability. Endothelial dysfunction facilitates the entry of low-density lipoprotein (LDL) cholesterol into the arterial wall and promotes leukocyte adhesion and transmigration, initiating the formation of atherosclerotic lesions.

- Dyslipidemia: Insulin resistance is associated with atherogenic dyslipidemia, characterized by elevated triglycerides, decreased high-density lipoprotein (HDL) cholesterol, and an increased proportion of small, dense LDL particles. Dyslipidemia promotes lipid accumulation, foam cell formation, and plaque progression in the arterial intima.

- Inflammation and Oxidative Stress: Insulin resistance induces a chronic inflammatory state characterized by increased production of pro-inflammatory cytokines, chemokines, and acute-phase reactants. Inflammatory mediators activate endothelial cells, macrophages, and vascular smooth muscle cells, leading to oxidative stress, foam cell formation, and plaque instability.

2. Clinical Implications:

- Cardiovascular Events: Insulin resistance serves as a major risk factor for cardiovascular events, including myocardial infarction, stroke, and peripheral artery disease. Individuals with insulin resistance are more likely to develop obstructive coronary artery disease and experience adverse cardiovascular outcomes compared to those without insulin resistance.

- Progression to Diabetes: Insulin resistance precedes the development of type 2 diabetes mellitus, a major risk factor for cardiovascular disease. Approximately 70-80% of individuals with type 2 diabetes have concomitant insulin resistance, further exacerbating their cardiovascular risk profile.

- Therapeutic Considerations: Targeting insulin resistance through lifestyle modifications, pharmacotherapy, and insulin-sensitizing agents may help mitigate the risk of hypertension and arteriosclerosis and improve cardiovascular outcomes. Antihypertensive medications, statins, and antiplatelet agents are commonly used to manage hypertension and prevent atherosclerotic complications in individuals with insulin resistance.

The correlation between insulin resistance,

hypertension, and arteriosclerosis underscores the complex interplay between metabolic and cardiovascular health. Insulin resistance serves as a common denominator linking these interconnected pathways, contributing to the development and progression of cardiovascular disease. Recognizing the role of insulin resistance in hypertension and arteriosclerosis is essential for risk stratification, early intervention, and targeted therapeutic approaches aimed at reducing the burden of cardiovascular morbidity and mortality. By addressing insulin resistance as a modifiable risk factor, healthcare providers can optimize cardiovascular outcomes and improve the overall health and well-being of individuals at risk for cardiovascular disease.

THE ROLE OF SUGAR AND REFINED CARBOHYDRATES:

Insulin Resistance

◆ ◆ ◆

In recent years, the consumption of sugar and refined carbohydrates has surged, paralleling the rise in insulin resistance and related metabolic disorders globally. This chapter delves into the intricate relationship between sugar, refined carbohydrates, and insulin resistance, exploring the underlying mechanisms, epidemiological evidence, and public health implications of excessive consumption of these dietary components.

Understanding Sugar and Refined Carbohydrates:

1. Sugar: Sugar, primarily in the form of sucrose (table sugar) and high-fructose corn syrup (HFCS), is ubiquitous in the modern diet, found

in sweetened beverages, desserts, snacks, and processed foods. Excessive sugar consumption contributes to caloric excess, dysregulation of glucose metabolism, and metabolic disturbances associated with insulin resistance.

2.	Refined	Carbohydrates:	Refined carbohydrates, including white flour, white rice, and processed grains, undergo extensive processing that removes fiber, vitamins, and minerals, resulting in a rapid spike in blood glucose levels upon consumption. Refined carbohydrate-rich foods such as white bread, pasta, and pastries are staples of the Western diet but are associated with insulin resistance and metabolic dysfunction.

Mechanisms Linking Sugar and Refined Carbohydrates to Insulin Resistance:

1. Glycemic Index and Load: Sugar and refined carbohydrates have high glycemic index (GI) and glycemic load (GL), leading to rapid spikes in blood glucose levels and subsequent hyperinsulinemia. Chronic exposure to high GI/GL foods promotes insulin resistance, pancreatic beta-cell dysfunction, and impaired glucose tolerance.

2. Lipogenesis and Hepatic Insulin Resistance: Excessive sugar intake contributes to de novo lipogenesis (DNL), the conversion of glucose to fatty acids in the liver. Elevated triglyceride

levels and hepatic fat accumulation impair insulin signaling pathways, leading to hepatic insulin resistance and dyslipidemia.

3. Fructose Metabolism: Fructose, a component of sucrose and HFCS, is metabolized primarily in the liver, where it promotes lipogenesis, uric acid production, and mitochondrial dysfunction. Chronic fructose consumption induces insulin resistance, visceral adiposity, and systemic inflammation, contributing to the development of metabolic syndrome.

4. Advanced Glycation End Products (AGEs): Sugar and refined carbohydrates undergo non-enzymatic glycation reactions with proteins, lipids, and nucleic acids, forming advanced glycation end products (AGEs). AGEs accumulate in tissues, leading to oxidative stress, inflammation, and endothelial dysfunction, all of which contribute to insulin resistance and vascular complications.

Epidemiological Evidence:

1. Sugar Consumption and Diabetes Risk: Epidemiological studies have consistently demonstrated a positive association between sugar consumption and the risk of type 2 diabetes mellitus. High intake of sugar-sweetened beverages, in particular, is linked to an increased risk of developing insulin resistance, obesity, and

metabolic syndrome.

2. Refined Carbohydrates and Metabolic Disorders: Longitudinal cohort studies have shown that diets high in refined carbohydrates are associated with an elevated risk of insulin resistance, cardiovascular diseases, and all-cause mortality. Conversely, diets rich in whole grains, fruits, and vegetables are inversely associated with insulin resistance and metabolic syndrome prevalence.

Public Health Implications:

1. Obesity Epidemic: Excessive consumption of sugar and refined carbohydrates contributes to the global obesity epidemic, which is closely intertwined with insulin resistance and related metabolic disorders. Obesity increases the risk of developing type 2 diabetes, hypertension, dyslipidemia, and cardiovascular diseases, exacerbating the burden on healthcare systems worldwide.

2. Policy Interventions: Public health initiatives aimed at reducing sugar and refined carbohydrate consumption include sugar taxes, front-of-package labeling, restrictions on marketing to children, and educational campaigns promoting healthy dietary patterns. Regulation of food environments, school meal programs, and food industry practices is essential to create supportive

environments for healthier eating habits.

3. Nutrition Education: Empowering individuals with evidence-based nutrition education and skills to make informed dietary choices is crucial in preventing and managing insulin resistance and related metabolic conditions. Promoting whole foods, fiber-rich carbohydrates, and mindful eating practices fosters dietary patterns that support metabolic health and reduce the risk of chronic diseases.

4. Role of Healthcare Providers: Healthcare providers play a pivotal role in screening, diagnosing, and managing insulin resistance and metabolic disorders in clinical settings. Integrating nutrition counseling, lifestyle interventions, and pharmacotherapy into routine care helps optimize patient outcomes and reduce the progression of insulin resistance to type 2 diabetes and cardiovascular diseases.

The pervasive influence of sugar and refined carbohydrates on insulin resistance underscores the importance of addressing dietary factors in the prevention and management of metabolic disorders. By understanding the mechanisms linking sugar and refined carbohydrates to insulin resistance, advocating for evidence-based dietary guidelines, and implementing public health interventions, we can mitigate the impact of excessive sugar consumption on global health.

Empowering individuals and communities to make healthier dietary choices is essential in curbing the rising tide of insulin resistance and its associated complications, promoting a future of metabolic wellness and vitality.

SUGAR AND CARBOHYDRATES CHRONIC KIDNEY DISEASE AND FATTY LIVER:

Unveiling the Sweet Threat

"Fasting is a sacred practice that reminds us of our resilience, our interconnectedness with nature, and the infinite capacity for transformation within ourselves."

Sugar and carbohydrate-rich foods have become staples of modern diets, contributing to the rising prevalence of chronic kidney disease (CKD) and non-alcoholic fatty liver disease (NAFLD) worldwide. The excessive consumption of sugar and carbohydrates not only leads to metabolic disturbances but also plays a significant role in the pathogenesis and progression of these debilitating conditions. This chapter delves into the intricate relationship between sugar, carbohydrates, CKD, and fatty liver, exploring the underlying mechanisms, epidemiological evidence, and clinical implications of their interplay.

Understanding Chronic Kidney Disease (CKD) and Fatty Liver Disease:

1. Chronic Kidney Disease (CKD): CKD is a progressive condition characterized by the gradual loss of kidney function over time, leading to impaired filtration and excretion of waste products and toxins. Common risk factors for CKD include hypertension, diabetes, obesity, and metabolic syndrome.

2. Non-alcoholic Fatty Liver Disease (NAFLD): NAFLD encompasses a spectrum of liver disorders ranging from simple hepatic steatosis (fatty liver) to non-alcoholic steatohepatitis (NASH), fibrosis, cirrhosis, and hepatocellular carcinoma. NAFLD is closely associated with insulin resistance, obesity, dyslipidemia, and metabolic syndrome.

The Impact of Sugar and Carbohydrates on Chronic Kidney Disease (CKD):

1. Glucose and Fructose Metabolism:

- Hyperglycemia: Excessive consumption of sugar and high-glycemic carbohydrates contributes to hyperglycemia, a hallmark of diabetes and metabolic syndrome. Prolonged exposure to high blood glucose levels damages the kidneys' filtration units (glomeruli) and renal tubules, leading to diabetic nephropathy and CKD progression.

- Fructose Metabolism: Fructose, a component of sucrose and high-fructose corn syrup (HFCS), is metabolized primarily in the liver, where it promotes lipogenesis, hepatic insulin resistance, and uric acid production. Elevated uric acid levels contribute to renal inflammation, oxidative stress, and renal endothelial dysfunction, exacerbating kidney injury in individuals with CKD.

2. Insulin Resistance and Metabolic Syndrome:

- Insulin Resistance: Sugar and refined carbohydrates induce insulin resistance, a key pathophysiological mechanism underlying metabolic syndrome and its complications, including CKD. Insulin resistance promotes dyslipidemia, hypertension, inflammation, and oxidative stress, all of which contribute to renal injury and progressive kidney dysfunction.

- Dyslipidemia: High-carbohydrate diets, particularly those rich in refined carbohydrates, contribute to dyslipidemia characterized by elevated triglycerides, decreased high-density lipoprotein (HDL) cholesterol, and increased small, dense low-density lipoprotein (LDL) particles. Dyslipidemia exacerbates renal lipid accumulation, glomerular injury, and interstitial fibrosis in CKD.

3. Advanced Glycation End Products (AGEs):

- Formation of AGEs: Sugar and carbohydrates undergo non-enzymatic glycation reactions with proteins, lipids, and nucleic acids, forming advanced glycation end products (AGEs). AGE accumulation in the kidney promotes renal inflammation, oxidative stress, and extracellular matrix deposition, contributing to glomerulosclerosis and tubulointerstitial fibrosis in CKD.

- Renal Consequences: AGEs activate pro-inflammatory pathways, including nuclear factor-kappa B (NF-κB) and transforming growth factor-beta (TGF-β), leading to the production of pro-fibrotic cytokines, chemokines, and matrix metalloproteinases. AGE-induced renal damage accelerates CKD progression and increases the risk of end-stage renal disease (ESRD).

The Impact of Sugar and Carbohydrates on Fatty Liver Disease:

1. Hepatic Lipid Accumulation:

- De Novo Lipogenesis (DNL): Excessive consumption of sugar and high-carbohydrate diets promotes de novo lipogenesis (DNL), the conversion of glucose to fatty acids in the liver. Elevated insulin levels and hyperglycemia stimulate DNL, leading to hepatic triglyceride accumulation and steatosis in NAFLD.

- Fructose Metabolism: Fructose metabolism in the liver promotes lipogenesis, triglyceride synthesis, and lipid droplet formation through activation of carbohydrate response element-binding protein (ChREBP) and sterol regulatory element-binding protein-1c (SREBP-1c) pathways. Fructose-induced lipogenesis contributes to hepatic steatosis and insulin resistance in NAFLD.

2. Insulin Resistance and Hepatic Inflammation:

- Insulin Resistance: Sugar and refined carbohydrates contribute to hepatic insulin resistance, characterized by impaired suppression of hepatic glucose production and increased lipogenesis. Hepatic insulin resistance promotes dyslipidemia, inflammation, and oxidative stress, exacerbating liver injury and fibrosis in NAFLD.

- Inflammatory Pathways: Insulin resistance and hepatic lipid accumulation activate inflammatory pathways, including c-Jun N-terminal kinase (JNK), toll-like receptor 4 (TLR4), and nuclear factor-kappa B (NF-κB), leading to the production of pro-inflammatory cytokines, such as tumor necrosis factor-alpha (TNF-α) and interleukin-6 (IL-6). Chronic inflammation promotes hepatocyte injury, immune cell infiltration, and activation of hepatic stellate cells, culminating in fibrosis and progression to advanced stages of NAFLD, including NASH and cirrhosis.

3. Gut-Liver Axis Dysfunction:

- Dysbiosis: Excessive consumption of sugar and carbohydrates alters the composition and diversity of the gut microbiota, leading to dysbiosis—a state of microbial imbalance characterized by overgrowth of pathogenic bacteria and depletion of beneficial microbes. Dysbiosis promotes gut permeability, bacterial translocation, and release of pro-inflammatory bacterial products, such as lipopolysaccharides (LPS), into the systemic circulation.

- Endotoxemia: LPS from gram-negative bacteria activate TLR4 signaling in hepatic Kupffer cells and immune cells, triggering the production of pro-inflammatory cytokines and reactive oxygen species (ROS). Chronic endotoxemia and low-grade systemic inflammation contribute to hepatic insulin resistance, lipid accumulation, and liver injury in NAFLD.

Clinical Implications and Management Strategies:

1. Dietary Modifications:

- Limit Sugar and Refined Carbohydrates: Restricting the intake of sugar-sweetened beverages, desserts, snacks, and processed foods high in refined carbohydrates is essential in preventing and managing CKD and fatty liver disease. Emphasizing whole foods, fiber-rich carbohydrates, and healthy fats promotes metabolic health and reduces the risk of metabolic complications.

- Mediterranean Diet: Adopting a Mediterranean-style diet rich in fruits, vegetables, legumes, nuts, whole grains, fish, and olive oil has been associated with improved renal function, reduced liver fat accumulation, and decreased risk of CKD and NAFLD. The Mediterranean diet emphasizes nutrient-dense, anti-inflammatory foods that support cardiovascular and metabolic health.

2. Lifestyle Interventions:

- Weight Management: Achieving and maintaining a healthy body weight through regular physical activity, calorie control, and portion moderation is essential in reducing the risk of obesity-related complications, including CKD and fatty liver disease. Lifestyle modifications that promote energy balance, such as aerobic exercise, resistance training, and mindful eating, improve insulin sensitivity and metabolic health.

- Smoking Cessation: Smoking is a modifiable

risk factor for CKD and liver disease, as it promotes inflammation, oxidative stress, and endothelial dysfunction. Smoking cessation reduces the risk of CKD progression, cardiovascular events, and liver fibrosis in individuals with NAFLD.

3. Pharmacological Interventions:

- Antihypertensive Therapy: Individuals with CKD and hypertension benefit from antihypertensive medications, such as angiotensin-converting enzyme (ACE) inhibitors and angiotensin II receptor blockers (ARBs), which improve renal hemodynamics, reduce proteinuria, and slow the progression of CKD. Blood pressure control is essential in preserving renal function and preventing cardiovascular complications.

- Insulin Sensitizers: Insulin-sensitizing agents, including metformin, thiazolidinediones, and glucagon-like peptide-1 (GLP-1) receptor agonists, improve insulin sensitivity, glycemic control, and hepatic lipid metabolism in individuals with NAFLD and insulin resistance. These medications reduce hepatic steatosis, inflammation, and fibrosis, and may be considered in patients with metabolic comorbidities.

4. Screening and Monitoring:

- Routine Screening: Healthcare providers should screen individuals at risk for CKD and NAFLD, including those with diabetes, hypertension, obesity, and metabolic syndrome, using laboratory tests, imaging studies, and clinical assessments. Early detection and intervention are crucial in preventing disease progression and improving long-term outcomes.

- Biomarkers: Novel biomarkers of renal function and liver injury, such as urinary albumin-to-creatinine ratio (ACR), estimated glomerular filtration rate (eGFR), liver enzymes (ALT, AST), and imaging modalities (ultrasound, MRI, transient elastography), aid in risk stratification, diagnosis, and monitoring of CKD and NAFLD. Biomarker panels reflecting inflammation, fibrosis, and oxidative stress provide insights into disease severity and prognosis.

The impact of sugar and carbohydrates on chronic kidney disease and fatty liver disease underscores the importance of dietary interventions, lifestyle modifications, and pharmacological therapies in mitigating the risk of metabolic complications and improving long-term outcomes. By understanding the complex interplay between dietary factors, metabolic dysregulation, and organ-specific pathology, healthcare providers can implement comprehensive management strategies tailored to individual needs and risk profiles. Empowering individuals with knowledge and resources to make informed dietary choices and lifestyle changes is essential in promoting metabolic health and preventing the progression of chronic kidney disease and fatty liver disease.

RELATIONSHIP BETWEEN SUGAR AND PANCREATIC CANCER:

Exposing the Sweet Menace

◆ ◆ ◆

Pancreatic cancer, one of the deadliest malignancies, poses a significant public health challenge due to its aggressive nature, limited treatment options, and poor prognosis. While several risk factors contribute to the development of pancreatic cancer, emerging evidence suggests a complex interplay between dietary factors, particularly sugar consumption, and pancreatic carcinogenesis. This chapter explores the intricate relationship between sugar and pancreatic cancer, elucidating the underlying mechanisms, epidemiological findings, and clinical implications of their association.

Understanding Pancreatic Cancer:

1. Pancreatic Cancer: Pancreatic cancer arises from the abnormal growth of cells in the pancreas, a vital organ responsible for producing digestive enzymes and hormones, including insulin and glucagon. Pancreatic tumors can originate from exocrine cells, forming adenocarcinomas, or endocrine cells, resulting in neuroendocrine tumors.

2. Risk Factors: Several risk factors contribute to the development of pancreatic cancer, including age, smoking, obesity, family history, chronic pancreatitis, and genetic predisposition (e.g., BRCA mutations, familial pancreatic cancer syndromes).

The Role of Sugar in Pancreatic Carcinogenesis:

1. Glucose Metabolism:

- Hyperglycemia: Excessive sugar consumption contributes to hyperglycemia—a state of elevated blood glucose levels—by overwhelming pancreatic beta cells' capacity to secrete insulin and maintain glucose homeostasis. Chronic hyperglycemia promotes pancreatic inflammation, oxidative stress, and oncogenic signaling pathways implicated in cancer initiation and progression.

- Insulin Resistance: Sugar-rich diets induce insulin resistance—a condition characterized by impaired insulin signaling and reduced cellular responsiveness to insulin—which leads to compensatory hyperinsulinemia and increased insulin-like growth factor 1 (IGF-1) levels. Insulin resistance promotes pancreatic carcinogenesis through mitogenic, pro-survival, and anti-apoptotic effects on cancer cells.

2. Inflammation and Oxidative Stress:

- Pro-inflammatory Effects: High-sugar diets contribute to systemic inflammation, adipose tissue inflammation, and release of pro-inflammatory cytokines, such as interleukin-6 (IL-6) and tumor necrosis factor-alpha (TNF-α). Chronic inflammation in the pancreas promotes oncogenic transformation, DNA damage, and tumor microenvironment remodeling conducive to tumor growth and metastasis.

- Oxidative Stress: Sugar metabolism generates reactive oxygen species (ROS) and free radicals, leading to oxidative damage to cellular components, including DNA, proteins, and lipids. Oxidative stress disrupts cellular redox balance, activates oncogenic signaling pathways, and promotes genetic instability in pancreatic cells, predisposing them to malignant transformation.

3. Insulin-like Growth Factor 1 (IGF-1) Signaling:

- Growth Promotion: Sugar consumption

stimulates insulin and IGF-1 signaling pathways, which play key roles in cell growth, proliferation, and survival. Elevated IGF-1 levels activate phosphatidylinositol 3-kinase (PI3K)/Akt and mitogen-activated protein kinase (MAPK) pathways, promoting cell cycle progression, angiogenesis, and resistance to apoptosis in pancreatic cancer cells.

- Tumor Progression: Dysregulated IGF-1 signaling promotes epithelial-mesenchymal transition (EMT), invasion, and metastasis in pancreatic cancer, contributing to tumor aggressiveness and therapeutic resistance. Targeting the IGF-1 axis represents a promising therapeutic strategy for inhibiting pancreatic cancer growth and metastatic spread.

Epidemiological Evidence:

1. Sugar Consumption and Pancreatic Cancer Risk:

- Prospective Cohort Studies: Epidemiological studies have demonstrated a positive association between high sugar intake, particularly from sugar-sweetened beverages (SSBs) and high-glycemic index (GI) foods, and an increased risk of pancreatic cancer. Individuals consuming large quantities of added sugars, fructose, and refined carbohydrates exhibit higher pancreatic cancer incidence rates compared to those with lower sugar intake.

- Meta-Analyses: Meta-analyses of observational studies have confirmed the link between sugar consumption and pancreatic cancer risk, highlighting the dose-response relationship between sugar intake, glycemic load, and pancreatic cancer incidence. Pooled analyses support the hypothesis that dietary sugars, independent of obesity and diabetes, contribute to pancreatic carcinogenesis through metabolic and inflammatory pathways.

2. Mechanistic Insights:

- Preclinical Models: Animal studies and cell culture experiments provide mechanistic insights into the oncogenic effects of sugar metabolism on pancreatic cells, elucidating the role of hyperglycemia, insulin resistance, inflammation, and IGF-1 signaling in promoting tumor initiation, progression, and metastasis. Preclinical models recapitulate the tumor-promoting effects of high-sugar diets, underscoring the relevance of dietary interventions in pancreatic cancer prevention and treatment.

Clinical Implications and Recommendations:

1. Dietary Modifications:

- Sugar Reduction: Limiting the consumption of added sugars, SSBs, sugary snacks, and processed foods high in refined carbohydrates is essential in reducing pancreatic cancer risk and improving metabolic health. Emphasizing whole foods, fiber-rich carbohydrates, and low-glycemic index options supports dietary patterns associated with reduced inflammation and cancer prevention.

-        Mediterranean Diet: Adopting a Mediterranean-style diet rich in fruits, vegetables, whole grains, fish, olive oil, and nuts offers protective benefits against pancreatic cancer by providing anti-inflammatory, antioxidant, and anti-carcinogenic compounds. The Mediterranean diet emphasizes plant-based foods, lean protein sources, and healthy fats that support overall health and reduce cancer risk.

2. Lifestyle Modifications:

- Weight Management: Maintaining a healthy body weight through regular physical activity, portion control, and calorie moderation reduces the risk of obesity-related cancers, including pancreatic cancer. Physical exercise, such as aerobic exercise, strength training, and flexibility exercises, enhances metabolic health, insulin sensitivity, and immune function, reducing cancer susceptibility.

- Smoking Cessation: Smoking cessation is paramount in pancreatic cancer prevention, as tobacco smoking is a major risk factor for pancreatic cancer development. Quitting smoking reduces exposure to carcinogens, inflammatory compounds, and oxidative stressors, decreasing the likelihood of pancreatic tumor initiation and progression.

3. Public Health Initiatives:

-   Nutrition Education: Public health campaigns and educational initiatives aimed at raising awareness about the detrimental effects of sugar consumption on pancreatic health and cancer risk are crucial in promoting dietary behavior change and reducing sugar-related pancreatic cancer incidence. Targeted messaging, nutritional counseling, and community-based interventions can empower individuals to make informed dietary choices, prioritize whole foods, and reduce their reliance on sugary beverages and processed snacks.

- Food Policy Interventions: Governmental regulations and food policies that promote healthier dietary environments, such as taxation on sugary drinks, front-of-package labeling, and restrictions on marketing unhealthy foods to children, play a pivotal role in shaping consumer behavior and reducing sugar consumption at the population level. Implementing evidence-based strategies to curb sugar intake aligns with public health efforts to prevent chronic diseases, including pancreatic cancer.

4. Early Detection and Screening:

- High-Risk Groups: Individuals with a family history of pancreatic cancer, hereditary cancer syndromes (e.g., BRCA mutations, Lynch syndrome), or certain predisposing conditions (e.g., chronic pancreatitis, diabetes) may benefit from early detection and surveillance programs. Identifying high-risk groups enables targeted screening efforts and proactive management strategies to detect pancreatic lesions at early, potentially curable stages.

- Biomarker Development: Advancements in biomarker research hold promise for improving early detection and risk stratification in pancreatic cancer. Biomarkers of sugar metabolism, inflammation, and pancreatic ductal changes may serve as non-invasive tools for identifying individuals at increased risk of pancreatic cancer and monitoring disease progression over time.

The relationship between sugar consumption and pancreatic cancer underscores the importance of dietary interventions, lifestyle modifications, and public health initiatives in reducing cancer risk and promoting pancreatic health. By understanding the molecular mechanisms linking sugar metabolism to pancreatic carcinogenesis, adopting healthy dietary patterns, and implementing evidence-based strategies for cancer prevention and early detection, we can mitigate the impact of sugar on pancreatic cancer incidence and improve overall population health. Empowering individuals, communities, and policymakers to prioritize sugar reduction initiatives and foster supportive environments for healthy eating is paramount in the fight against pancreatic cancer and other diet-related cancers. Through collaborative efforts and interdisciplinary approaches, we can pave the way for a future where pancreatic cancer incidence is minimized, and individuals thrive in environments conducive to optimal health and well-being.

NEUROLOGICAL DISEASES, DEMENTIA, AND ALZHEIMER'S:

Try not to forget this piece of knowledge.

◆ ◆ ◆

In recent years, mounting evidence has highlighted the detrimental impact of sugar consumption on brain health, implicating it as a potential risk factor for neurological diseases, dementia, and Alzheimer's disease (AD). This chapter delves into the intricate relationship between sugar and neurodegenerative disorders, elucidating the underlying mechanisms, epidemiological findings, and clinical implications of their association.

Understanding Neurological Diseases, Dementia, and Alzheimer's:

1. Neurological Diseases: Neurological diseases encompass a broad spectrum of disorders affecting the central and peripheral nervous systems, including neurodegenerative conditions, movement disorders, epilepsy, stroke, and neurodevelopmental disorders.

2. Dementia: Dementia refers to a progressive decline in cognitive function and memory, characterized by impairments in reasoning, language, visuospatial skills, and executive function. Alzheimer's disease is the most common cause of dementia, accounting for the majority of cases worldwide.

3. Alzheimer's Disease (AD): Alzheimer's disease is a neurodegenerative disorder characterized by the accumulation of amyloid-beta plaques and tau tangles in the brain, leading to neuronal loss, synaptic dysfunction, and cognitive decline. AD is the leading cause of dementia in older adults, affecting millions of individuals globally.

The Impact of Sugar on Neurological Health:

1. Glycemic Dysregulation:

- Hyperglycemia: Excessive sugar consumption contributes to hyperglycemia, insulin resistance, and dysregulation of glucose metabolism, all of which are implicated in the pathogenesis of neurological diseases and cognitive impairment.

- Insulin Resistance: Insulin resistance in the brain impairs insulin signaling pathways, disrupts glucose uptake and utilization by neurons, and promotes neuroinflammation, oxidative stress, and synaptic dysfunction.

- Glucose Excitotoxicity: Prolonged exposure to high glucose levels exacerbates excitotoxicity—a process involving excessive release of excitatory neurotransmitters, such as glutamate, leading to neuronal injury, apoptosis, and cognitive deficits.

2. Neuroinflammation and Oxidative Stress:

- Pro-inflammatory Effects: Sugar consumption promotes systemic inflammation and crosses the blood-brain barrier, activating microglia—the resident immune cells of the central nervous system. Chronic neuroinflammation contributes to neurodegeneration, synaptic dysfunction, and cognitive decline in neurological diseases.

- Oxidative Stress: Sugar metabolism generates reactive oxygen species (ROS) and free radicals, leading to oxidative damage to neuronal membranes, proteins, and DNA. Oxidative stress accelerates aging-related changes in the brain and increases the risk of neurodegenerative disorders, including AD.

3. Advanced Glycation End Products (AGEs):

- Formation of AGEs: Sugar and its metabolites undergo non-enzymatic glycation reactions with proteins, lipids, and nucleic acids, forming advanced glycation end products (AGEs). AGE accumulation in the brain promotes neuroinflammation, tau hyperphosphorylation, and amyloid-beta aggregation, contributing to AD pathogenesis.

- Cross-linking and Protein Aggregation: AGEs cross-link structural proteins, impair enzymatic activity, and promote protein aggregation, leading to the formation of neurofibrillary tangles and amyloid plaques—hallmarks of AD pathology.

Epidemiological Evidence:

1. Sugar Consumption and Cognitive Decline:

- Longitudinal Studies: Epidemiological studies have shown a positive association between high sugar intake and cognitive decline, dementia, and AD risk in older adults. Excessive consumption of sugar-sweetened beverages, desserts, and processed foods is linked to poorer cognitive performance and accelerated brain aging.

- Framingham Heart Study: Participants with higher dietary glycemic index (GI) and glycemic load (GL) scores had an increased risk of cognitive impairment and dementia over a 6-year follow-up period, independent of other dietary and lifestyle factors.

- Rotterdam Study: High intake of sugar-sweetened beverages was associated with an elevated risk of incident dementia and AD in a large cohort of older adults, highlighting the detrimental effects of sugar on brain health.

2. Metabolic Syndrome and Cognitive Dysfunction:

- Shared Risk Factors: Metabolic syndrome —a cluster of interconnected metabolic abnormalities including obesity, hypertension, dyslipidemia, and insulin resistance—is associated with an increased risk of cognitive dysfunction, vascular dementia, and AD. Sugar consumption contributes to the development of metabolic syndrome and exacerbates cognitive impairment through neuroinflammatory and neurodegenerative mechanisms.

- Bidirectional Relationship: Cognitive impairment and dementia, in turn, exacerbate metabolic dysfunction, creating a vicious cycle of cognitive decline and metabolic dysregulation. Addressing modifiable risk factors, including sugar consumption, is essential in preventing or delaying the onset of cognitive decline and neurodegenerative diseases.

Clinical Implications and Recommendations:

1. Dietary Modifications:

- Mediterranean Diet: Adopting a Mediterranean-style diet rich in fruits, vegetables, whole grains, nuts, seeds, fish, and olive oil has been associated with improved cognitive function, reduced risk of dementia, and slower progression of AD. The Mediterranean diet emphasizes anti-inflammatory foods, antioxidants, and healthy fats that support brain health and cognitive resilience.

- Low-Glycemic Diet: Limiting the consumption of high-glycemic carbohydrates, sugary snacks, and processed foods helps stabilize blood glucose levels, reduce insulin resistance, and mitigate the risk of cognitive decline and neurodegenerative disorders. Choosing fiber-rich carbohydrates, such as legumes, whole grains, and non-starchy vegetables, promotes satiety, glycemic control, and brain health.

2. Lifestyle Interventions:

- Physical Activity: Regular physical exercise improves cerebral blood flow, neuroplasticity, and cognitive function, reducing the risk of cognitive decline and dementia. Aerobic exercise, resistance training, and mind-body practices, such as yoga and tai chi, enhance brain health and mitigate the deleterious effects of sugar on neurological function.

- Cognitive Stimulation: Engaging in mentally stimulating activities, such as reading, puzzles, learning new skills, and social interaction, preserves cognitive function and promotes neurogenesis—a process of generating new neurons and synaptic connections in the brain. Cognitive enrichment enhances cognitive reserve and resilience against age-related cognitive decline and neurodegenerative diseases.

3. Blood Sugar Monitoring:

- Glycemic Control: Individuals at risk for cognitive impairment and neurodegenerative diseases should monitor their blood sugar levels regularly, maintain glycemic control, and seek medical advice if glucose levels are consistently elevated. Lifestyle modifications, medication adherence, and glucose-lowering therapies help mitigate the neurotoxic effects of hyperglycemia on the brain.

- Continuous Glucose Monitoring (CGM): CGM devices provide real-time glucose monitoring and feedback, enabling individuals to track their dietary choices, physical activity levels, and glucose responses throughout the day. CGM technology facilitates personalized interventions and behavioral modifications to optimize glycemic control and brain health.

4. Neuroprotective Supplements:

- Omega-3 Fatty Acids: Omega-3 polyunsaturated fatty acids, found in fatty fish, flaxseeds, and walnuts, exert neuroprotective effects by reducing neuroinflammation, oxidative stress, and synaptic dysfunction. Omega-3 supplementation may improve cognitive function and attenuate neurodegeneration in individuals at risk for dementia and AD.

- Antioxidants: Antioxidant-rich foods, such as berries, dark chocolate, green tea, and colorful fruits and vegetables, contain phytochemicals that scavenge free radicals, mitigate oxidative damage, and enhance brain resilience. Antioxidant supplements, including vitamin E, vitamin C, and coenzyme Q10, may support cognitive health and delay age-related cognitive decline.

Conclusion:

Compelling evidence linking sugar consumption to neurological diseases, dementia, and Alzheimer's disease underscores the urgent need for public health interventions and individualized strategies to mitigate the impact of sugar on brain health. By understanding the neurobiological mechanisms underlying sugar-induced neurotoxicity, promoting dietary modifications, lifestyle interventions, and neuroprotective supplements, we can optimize cognitive function, preserve brain health, and reduce the burden of neurodegenerative disorders on individuals, families, and society. Empowering individuals with knowledge, resources, and support to make informed lifestyle choices is paramount in promoting brain resilience and enhancing quality of life across the lifespan.

GOVERNMENT'S ROLE PROMOTING A HIGH SUGAR AND CARBOHYDRATES DIET:

Assessing Policies, Industry Influence, and Public Health Implications

◆ ◆ ◆

The prevalence of high sugar and carbohydrates diets is a pressing public health concern, contributing to the global rise in obesity, diabetes, and other chronic diseases. While individual dietary choices play a significant role, governmental policies, food industry practices, and societal norms also influence consumption patterns. This chapter examines the government's role in promoting a high sugar and carbohydrates diet, exploring policy frameworks, industry regulations, and public health implications.

Government Policies and Regulations:

1. Dietary Guidelines:

- Nutritional Recommendations: Governmental agencies, such as the U.S. Department of Agriculture (USDA) and Health Canada, issue dietary guidelines that inform public health strategies and consumer behavior. Historically, dietary guidelines emphasized low-fat diets while paying less attention to sugar and carbohydrate intake, inadvertently promoting consumption of processed foods high in added sugars and refined carbohydrates.

- Evolving Guidelines: In recent years, dietary guidelines have evolved to address the adverse health effects of excessive sugar consumption and refined carbohydrate intake. Updated recommendations emphasize the importance of limiting added sugars, choosing whole grains over refined grains, and prioritizing nutrient-dense foods in the diet. However, implementation and enforcement of these guidelines vary across jurisdictions and may be influenced by political and industry interests.

2. Food Labeling and Nutrition Policies:

- Nutrition Labeling: Government-mandated nutrition labeling requirements provide consumers with information about the sugar and carbohydrate content of packaged foods and beverages. However, labeling regulations may not adequately reflect the contribution of added sugars to total carbohydrate content, leading to confusion among consumers and underestimation of sugar intake.

- Front-of-Package Labeling: Some governments have implemented front-of-package labeling systems to help consumers make healthier food choices by highlighting nutritional attributes, such as sugar content, on food packaging. Traffic light labeling and interpretive symbols provide at-a-glance information about the nutritional quality of food products, empowering consumers to make informed decisions.

3. Agricultural Subsidies and Farm Policies:

- Crop Subsidies: Government agricultural policies, including crop subsidies and price supports, influence the production and availability of agricultural commodities, such as corn, wheat, and soybeans, which are major sources of sugars and refined carbohydrates in the food supply. Subsidies favoring commodity crops over fruits, vegetables, and whole grains may contribute to the prevalence of cheap, processed foods high in added sugars and low in nutritional value.

- Farm Bill: The U.S. Farm Bill, a comprehensive piece of legislation reauthorized every five years, shapes agricultural policy, nutrition assistance programs, and food industry practices. Critics argue that the Farm Bill prioritizes the interests of agribusiness and commodity producers over public health and environmental sustainability, perpetuating a food system that incentivizes the production and consumption of high-sugar, low-nutrient foods.

Industry Influence and Marketing Practices:

1. Food Industry Lobbying:

- Influence on Policy: The food industry wields considerable influence over government policies and regulatory decisions through lobbying efforts, campaign contributions, and industry-funded research. Lobbying by food and beverage manufacturers, trade associations, and industry groups may shape agricultural policies, nutrition programs, and public health initiatives to favor the interests of the industry over public health concerns.

- Regulatory Capture: Regulatory capture occurs when government agencies tasked with overseeing the food industry become influenced or controlled by industry interests, compromising their ability to enact and enforce evidence-based regulations. Revolving door dynamics between government agencies and industry positions may further entrench industry influence and undermine public health objectives.

2. Marketing to Children:

- Targeted Advertising: Food and beverage companies employ targeted marketing strategies to promote high-sugar and carbohydrate-rich products to children and adolescents through television, digital media, and social networking platforms. Branding, packaging, and product placement tactics influence children's preferences, consumption patterns, and dietary habits, contributing to the pervasive exposure to unhealthy foods in the media environment.

- Product Placement: Product placement in schools, sports events, and entertainment venues exposes children to marketing messages promoting sugary snacks, sugary beverages, and convenience foods as desirable choices for snacks, meals, and refreshments. Tie-ins with popular characters, movies, and television shows enhance brand recognition and appeal among young consumers, reinforcing associations between sugary products and positive experiences.

Public Health Implications and Challenges:

1. Rising Rates of Obesity and Chronic Diseases:

- Health Consequences: The government's

promotion of a high sugar and carbohydrates diet contributes to the obesity epidemic and the increasing prevalence of diet-related chronic diseases, including type 2 diabetes, cardiovascular diseases, and certain cancers. Excessive sugar consumption and refined carbohydrate intake are major drivers of weight gain, insulin resistance, and metabolic dysregulation, placing individuals at heightened risk of developing obesity-related comorbidities.

- Disparities in Health Outcomes: Socioeconomic and racial/ethnic disparities in diet-related health outcomes reflect inequities in access to healthy foods, nutrition education, and healthcare resources. Vulnerable populations, including low-income communities and communities of color, are disproportionately affected by the adverse health effects of high-sugar diets, experiencing higher rates of obesity, diabetes, and cardiovascular diseases.

2. Environmental Impact:

- Agricultural Practices: Intensive agricultural practices associated with the production of sugar crops, such as sugarcane and sugar beets, contribute to environmental degradation, deforestation, and biodiversity loss. Monocropping, chemical inputs, and water-intensive cultivation methods used in sugar production have adverse environmental impacts, including soil erosion, water pollution, and habitat destruction.

- Climate Change: The agricultural sector's reliance on fossil fuels, land use change, and deforestation for sugar production contributes to greenhouse gas emissions, climate change, and environmental degradation. Carbon-intensive agricultural practices, such as mechanized harvesting, irrigation, and transportation of sugar crops, exacerbate the carbon footprint of the food system, exacerbating climate-related risks and environmental challenges.

3. Policy Reform and Advocacy:

- Evidence-Based Interventions: Policymakers, public health advocates, and grassroots organizations advocate for evidence-based interventions to address the government's role in promoting a high sugar and carbohydrates diet and mitigate its adverse health effects. Policy reform efforts focus on implementing sugar taxes, restricting marketing to children, improving food labeling, and promoting sustainable agricultural practices to create environments conducive to healthier dietary choices.

- Multisectoral Collaboration: Collaborative approaches involving government agencies, public health organizations, civil society groups, and industry stakeholders are essential for implementing comprehensive strategies to promote healthier diets and reduce the consumption of high-sugar foods and beverages. Multisectoral collaboration facilitates coordination, resource mobilization, and collective action across diverse stakeholders to address complex public health challenges.

The government plays a significant role in shaping dietary patterns, food environments, and public health outcomes through its policies, regulations, and industry interactions. Efforts to address the government's promotion of a high sugar and carbohydrates diet require a multifaceted approach that addresses systemic drivers of poor nutrition, industry influence, and socioeconomic disparities in access to healthy foods. By prioritizing evidence-based interventions, fostering multisectoral collaboration, and advocating for policy reform, stakeholders can work together to create environments that support healthier dietary choices and improve population health outcomes. Through concerted action and sustained advocacy, we can build a healthier, more equitable food system that promotes well-being for all.

ADDICTION, SUGAR, AND CARBOHYDRATES:

Unveiling the Sweet Trap

"Food addiction: where the mind craves what the body doesn't need."

◆ ◆ ◆

In recent decades, the consumption of sugar and carbohydrates has skyrocketed, paralleling the rise in rates of obesity, diabetes, and metabolic disorders worldwide. Beyond their nutritional value, sugar and carbohydrates have been implicated in addictive behaviors, fueling debates about their role in driving excessive consumption and contributing to adverse health outcomes. This chapter delves into the intricate relationship between addiction, sugar, and carbohydrates, exploring the underlying mechanisms, behavioral aspects, and public health implications of this complex interplay.

Understanding Sugar and Carbohydrate Addiction:

1. Sugar Addiction: Sugar addiction refers to a pattern of compulsive, hedonically-driven consumption of sweet foods and beverages, characterized by cravings, tolerance, withdrawal symptoms, and loss of control over intake. While not formally recognized as a diagnosable disorder in the Diagnostic and Statistical Manual of Mental Disorders (DSM-5), sugar addiction shares similarities with substance use disorders in terms of neurobiology and behavioral manifestations.

2. Carbohydrate Addiction: Carbohydrate addiction encompasses a broader spectrum of refined carbohydrates, including white flour, white rice, and processed grains, which elicit rapid spikes in blood glucose levels and promote hedonic eating behaviors. Carbohydrate-rich foods such as bread, pasta, and pastries are commonly craved and consumed in excess by individuals with carbohydrate addiction.

Mechanisms Underlying Sugar and Carbohydrate Addiction:

1. Neurobiological Pathways:

   - Reward System Activation: Sugar and

refined carbohydrates activate the brain's reward system, including the mesolimbic dopamine pathway, leading to the release of dopamine —a neurotransmitter associated with pleasure and reinforcement. Chronic exposure to high-sugar, high-carbohydrate diets desensitize dopamine receptors, contributing to compulsive consumption and tolerance.

- Neurotransmitter Dysregulation: Sugar and carbohydrates influence other neurotransmitter systems involved in reward processing, including serotonin, opioids, and endocannabinoids. Dysregulated neurotransmitter signaling may contribute to mood disturbances, cravings, and addictive behaviors.

- Hypothalamic-Pituitary-Adrenal (HPA) Axis: Chronic sugar and carbohydrate consumption dysregulates the hypothalamic-pituitary-adrenal (HPA) axis, leading to alterations in stress hormone secretion, cortisol levels, and stress-induced eating behaviors. Stress-related eating may exacerbate addictive tendencies and promote overeating in response to emotional cues.

- Neuroinflammation: Sugar and refined carbohydrates contribute to neuroinflammation, characterized by increased production of pro-inflammatory cytokines, microglial activation, and oxidative stress in the brain. Neuroinflammation may disrupt neurotransmitter balance, impair reward circuitry function, and contribute to addictive behaviors.

2. Hedonic Eating Behaviors:

- Palatability and Hyperpalatability: Sugar and refined carbohydrates are highly palatable due to their sweet taste, smooth texture, and rapid absorption, which stimulate pleasure centers in the brain. Hyperpalatable foods, rich in sugar, fat, and salt, override satiety signals and promote overconsumption, contributing to addictive-like eating behaviors.

- Cravings and Withdrawal: Sugar and carbohydrate cravings are driven by physiological and psychological factors, including neurobiological adaptations, conditioned responses, and emotional triggers. Withdrawal symptoms, such as irritability, fatigue, and dysphoria, may occur upon cessation of sugar or carbohydrate intake, perpetuating addictive cycles.

Behavioral Aspects of Sugar and Carbohydrate Addiction:

1. Cue Reactivity and Conditioning:

- Environmental Cues: Sugar and carbohydrate addiction is influenced by environmental cues, such as food advertisements, availability, social norms, and cultural traditions. Exposure to food cues triggers conditioned responses, activates reward pathways, and increases the likelihood of consumption, even in the absence of hunger.

- Stress and Emotions: Stress, negative emotions, and psychological distress play a role in sugar and carbohydrate addiction, as individuals may seek comfort or distraction through emotional eating. Emotional dysregulation, coping mechanisms, and maladaptive stress responses contribute to addictive eating behaviors.

2. Sociocultural Influences:

- Food Marketing: The food industry employs sophisticated marketing strategies to promote sugary and carbohydrate-rich products, targeting vulnerable populations, including children, adolescents, and individuals with low socioeconomic status. Marketing tactics, such as product placement, celebrity endorsements, and persuasive advertising, shape consumer preferences and drive consumption patterns.

- Social Norms and Peer Pressure: Social norms surrounding food consumption, celebrations, and social gatherings influence dietary choices and eating behaviors. Peer pressure, social comparison, and social reinforcement may facilitate the adoption of unhealthy eating habits and exacerbate addictive tendencies.

Public Health Implications:

1. Obesity and Metabolic Disorders: Sugar and carbohydrate addiction contribute to the global obesity epidemic and the prevalence of metabolic disorders, including type 2 diabetes, cardiovascular diseases, and non-alcoholic fatty liver disease (NAFLD). Excessive consumption of high-energy, low-nutrient foods undermines efforts to maintain a balanced diet and healthy weight.

2. Policy Interventions: Public health initiatives aimed at curbing sugar and carbohydrate addiction include sugar taxes, front-of-package labeling, restrictions on marketing to children, and education campaigns promoting mindful eating habits. Regulation of food environments, school meal programs, and food industry practices is essential to promote healthier dietary patterns and reduce the burden of diet-related diseases.

3. Nutrition Education: Nutrition education programs targeting individuals, families, and communities play a crucial role in raising awareness about the addictive properties of sugar and refined carbohydrates, fostering informed food choices, and promoting dietary diversity and balance. Empowering individuals with knowledge and skills to resist food temptations and manage

cravings is essential for long-term behavior change.

The complex relationship between addiction, sugar, and carbohydrates underscores the need for comprehensive approaches to address the pervasive influence of highly palatable, hyperpalatable foods on dietary habits and health outcomes. By understanding the neurobiological, behavioral, and sociocultural factors driving sugar and carbohydrate addiction, public health stakeholders can develop targeted interventions to promote healthier eating behaviors, mitigate the impact of food addiction on chronic diseases, and improve population health and well-being. Empowering individuals to make informed choices and cultivate mindful eating habits is paramount in navigating the sweet trap of sugar and carbohydrate addiction and fostering a culture of health and resilience.

"Through fasting, we reclaim our sovereignty over food, reconnect with our intuition, and rediscover the innate wisdom of our bodies." - Unknown

HARNESSING THE POWER OF FASTING:

Exploring its Healing Abilities and Therapeutic Potential

"For the desires of the flesh are against the Spirit, and the desires of the Spirit are against the flesh, for these are opposed to each other, to keep you from doing the things you want to do." - Galatians 5:17 (ESV)

◆ ◆ ◆

Fasting, the voluntary abstinence from food and caloric beverages for a defined period, has been practiced for centuries for various cultural, religious, and health-related reasons. In recent years, scientific research has unveiled the profound physiological effects of fasting on the body, leading to a resurgence of interest in its therapeutic potential. This chapter delves into the power of fasting, exploring its healing abilities, physiological mechanisms, and therapeutic applications across different health conditions.

Understanding Fasting:

1. Types of Fasting:

- Intermittent Fasting (IF): IF involves cycling between periods of fasting and eating, typically on a daily or weekly basis. Popular IF protocols include the 16/8 method (fasting for 16 hours, eating within an 8-hour window), the 5:2 diet (eating normally for 5 days, restricting calories on 2 non-consecutive days), and alternate-day fasting (fasting every other day).

- Prolonged Fasting: Prolonged fasting refers to extended periods of fasting lasting 24 hours or more, often practiced for multiple days or weeks. Water fasting, juice fasting, and fasting-mimicking diets (FMDs) are examples of prolonged fasting regimens used for therapeutic purposes.

2. Physiological Responses to Fasting:

- Metabolic Switch: During fasting, the body transitions from glucose metabolism to fat metabolism, depleting glycogen stores and mobilizing fatty acids for energy production through beta-oxidation and ketogenesis. Ketone bodies, such as beta-hydroxybutyrate (BHB), serve as alternative fuel sources for the brain and tissues during fasting.

- Hormonal Changes: Fasting modulates hormone levels, including insulin, glucagon, growth hormone, and adiponectin, which regulate metabolism, energy balance, and cellular repair processes. Insulin sensitivity improves, promoting glucose uptake by cells and reducing blood glucose levels, while growth hormone secretion increases, stimulating fat breakdown and muscle preservation.

- Autophagy Activation: Fasting triggers autophagy—a cellular recycling process that removes damaged organelles, protein aggregates, and dysfunctional components, promoting cellular renewal, repair, and longevity. Autophagy plays a crucial role in maintaining cellular homeostasis, preventing oxidative stress, and enhancing resilience to stressors.

The Healing Abilities of Fasting:

1. Weight Loss and Metabolic Health:

- Fat Loss: Fasting promotes fat loss and facilitates weight management by creating a calorie deficit, enhancing lipolysis, and increasing metabolic rate through thermogenesis. IF regimens, such as time-restricted feeding and alternate-day fasting, are effective strategies for reducing body weight, visceral fat, and obesity-related comorbidities.

- Metabolic Syndrome: Fasting improves metabolic health markers, including insulin sensitivity, blood glucose levels, lipid profile, and blood pressure, reducing the risk of metabolic syndrome, type 2 diabetes, and cardiovascular diseases. Fasting regimens that incorporate dietary modifications and lifestyle interventions support sustainable weight loss and metabolic improvements.

2. Cellular Repair and Longevity:

- Autophagy Enhancement: Fasting-induced autophagy promotes cellular detoxification, repair, and regeneration, enhancing mitochondrial function, DNA repair, and proteostasis. Autophagy activation may delay aging-related decline, mitigate age-related diseases, and extend lifespan in model organisms and humans.

- Stem Cell Activation: Fasting stimulates the production and mobilization of stem cells, including hematopoietic stem cells (HSCs) and mesenchymal stem cells (MSCs), which contribute to tissue regeneration, wound healing, and tissue repair processes. Stem cell rejuvenation may enhance tissue resilience and repair capacity, promoting longevity and vitality.

3. Neuroprotection and Cognitive Health:

- Brain Health: Fasting exerts neuroprotective effects by enhancing synaptic plasticity, neurogenesis, and brain-derived neurotrophic factor (BDNF) expression, which support cognitive function, memory consolidation, and mood regulation. Fasting regimens have shown promise in mitigating neurodegenerative diseases, such as Alzheimer's disease, Parkinson's disease, and stroke.

- Cognitive Performance: Fasting improves cognitive performance, attention, and executive function through mechanisms involving increased BHB levels, enhanced mitochondrial biogenesis, and reduced neuroinflammation. Intermittent fasting may enhance brain resilience to oxidative stress, neurotoxic insults, and age-related cognitive decline.

Therapeutic Applications of Fasting:

1. Metabolic Disorders:

- Type 2 Diabetes: Fasting regimens, such as intermittent fasting and time-restricted feeding, improve glycemic control, insulin sensitivity, and pancreatic function in individuals with type 2 diabetes. Fasting-induced ketosis may reduce insulin requirements, lower fasting blood glucose levels, and promote weight loss in diabetic patients.

- Obesity: Fasting interventions are effective in combating obesity and metabolic syndrome by promoting fat loss, preserving lean mass, and regulating appetite hormones. Alternate-day fasting, periodic fasting, and fasting-mimicking diets offer sustainable weight loss strategies with metabolic benefits beyond calorie restriction alone.

2. Cardiovascular Health:

- Heart Disease: Fasting regimens support cardiovascular health by reducing risk factors for heart disease, including hypertension, dyslipidemia, inflammation, and oxidative stress. Intermittent fasting and periodic fasting may improve lipid profiles, blood pressure, endothelial function, and myocardial energetics, reducing the risk of atherosclerosis and coronary artery disease.

3. Neurological Disorders:

- Alzheimer's Disease: Fasting has emerged as a promising therapeutic approach for Alzheimer's disease, as it targets multiple pathogenic mechanisms, including amyloid-beta accumulation, tau hyperphosphorylation, neuroinflammation, and oxidative stress. Intermittent fasting, ketogenic diet, and calorie restriction mimic the benefits of fasting on brain health and cognitive function in preclinical and clinical studies.

- Parkinson's Disease: Fasting regimens show potential in mitigating Parkinson's disease symptoms, enhancing dopamine signaling, and promoting neuroprotection against dopaminergic neuron degeneration. Ketogenic diets and intermittent fasting may alleviate motor symptoms, improve mitochondrial function, and enhance quality of life in Parkinson's patients.

Fasting holds tremendous therapeutic potential for promoting healthspan, enhancing resilience, and preventing a myriad of chronic diseases by harnessing the body's innate regenerative capacity and adaptive responses to nutrient deprivation. Through metabolic adaptation, cellular repair, and neuroprotective mechanisms, fasting promotes holistic healing, rejuvenation, and optimization of physiological function. Further research is warranted to elucidate the optimal fasting protocols, individualized approaches, and long-term effects of fasting on human health, paving the way for personalized lifestyle interventions and integrative strategies to optimize well-being and vitality across the lifespan.

SCIENCE OF FAT ADAPTATION AND WEIGHT LOSS:

Exploring Mechanisms, Benefits, and Practical Strategies

"So we fasted and petitioned our God about this, and he answered our prayer." - Ezra 8:23 (NIV)

◆ ◆ ◆

In recent years, fat adaptation has emerged as a popular approach for weight loss and metabolic health improvement. Unlike conventional low-fat diets, which prioritize carbohydrate consumption, fat adaptation emphasizes the utilization of fat as the primary fuel source for energy production. This essay delves into the science behind fat adaptation and weight loss, elucidating the physiological mechanisms, potential benefits, and practical strategies for achieving metabolic flexibility and sustainable weight management.

Understanding Fat Adaptation:

1. Metabolic Flexibility:

- Fuel Substrate Utilization: Metabolic flexibility refers to the ability of the body to adapt its fuel substrate utilization in response to changes in nutrient availability and energy demands. Under normal physiological conditions, the body switches between glucose and fatty acids as primary energy substrates, depending on dietary composition, physical activity levels, and metabolic state.

- Shift to Fat Oxidation: Fat adaptation involves enhancing the capacity of skeletal muscle mitochondria to oxidize fatty acids for energy production, thereby reducing reliance on glucose and glycogen stores during prolonged fasting or low-carbohydrate intake. Fat-adapted individuals exhibit increased rates of fatty acid oxidation, ketone utilization, and preservation of glycogen stores, supporting sustained energy supply and metabolic homeostasis.

2. Ketogenic Metabolism:

- Ketone Production: Fat adaptation promotes the production of ketone bodies, such as beta-hydroxybutyrate (BHB), acetoacetate, and acetone, through hepatic ketogenesis from fatty acids derived from adipose tissue triglycerides and dietary fat intake. Ketone bodies serve as alternative energy substrates for tissues, including the brain, heart, and skeletal muscle, during periods of carbohydrate restriction or prolonged fasting.

- Ketosis: Ketosis, a metabolic state characterized by elevated circulating ketone levels, occurs when carbohydrate availability is limited, and hepatic glycogen stores are depleted. Nutritional ketosis achieved through carbohydrate restriction (<50 grams per day) induces metabolic adaptations favoring fat oxidation, ketone production, and ketone utilization, facilitating weight loss and metabolic improvements in obese and insulin-resistant individuals.

Physiological Mechanisms of Fat Adaptation:

1. Hormonal Regulation:

- Insulin Sensitivity: Fat adaptation enhances insulin sensitivity and glucose uptake in skeletal muscle cells, reducing insulin resistance and hyperinsulinemia associated with high-carbohydrate diets. Reduced carbohydrate intake and lower postprandial glucose levels promote downregulation of insulin secretion, facilitating lipolysis, fatty acid oxidation, and ketogenesis in adipose tissue and liver.

- Hormonal Signaling: Hormonal responses to fat adaptation include increased secretion of glucagon, growth hormone, and catecholamines, which promote lipolysis, mobilization of fatty acids from adipose tissue, and ketogenesis in the liver. Hormonal adaptations support metabolic flexibility, substrate switching, and energy balance regulation in response to nutrient availability and energy demands.

2. Mitochondrial Biogenesis:

- Mitochondrial Adaptations: Fat adaptation stimulates mitochondrial biogenesis, oxidative capacity, and efficiency in skeletal muscle cells, enhancing mitochondrial fatty acid oxidation and ATP production. Increased expression of mitochondrial enzymes, such as carnitine palmitoyltransferase-1 (CPT-1) and beta-oxidation enzymes, supports fatty acid transport into mitochondria and subsequent oxidation via the tricarboxylic acid (TCA) cycle and electron transport chain.

- Enhanced Energy Efficiency: Fat-adapted individuals demonstrate improved energy efficiency, as evidenced by lower respiratory exchange ratios (RERs) and higher fat oxidation rates during submaximal exercise. Shifts in substrate utilization from carbohydrates to fats result in greater reliance on fat-derived fuels, preservation of glycogen stores, and delayed onset of fatigue during prolonged endurance activities.

Benefits of Fat Adaptation for Weight Loss:

1. Increased Fat Oxidation:

- Enhanced Fat Loss: Fat adaptation promotes increased fat oxidation rates and utilization of stored adipose tissue triglycerides for energy production, facilitating fat loss and body composition improvements in overweight and obese individuals. Compared to low-fat diets, which rely predominantly on glucose metabolism, fat-adapted individuals exhibit greater mobilization and oxidation of stored fat reserves, leading to more significant reductions in body fat mass.

- Appetite Regulation: Ketogenic diets and fat adaptation promote satiety, appetite suppression, and reduced caloric intake through hormonal and metabolic mechanisms. Ketone bodies, particularly beta-hydroxybutyrate (BHB), suppress appetite-regulating hormones, such as ghrelin, and increase levels of satiety hormones, such as cholecystokinin (CCK) and peptide YY (PYY), leading to decreased hunger and improved adherence to caloric restriction.

2. Stable Blood Glucose Levels:

- Improved Glycemic Control: Fat adaptation improves glycemic control and stabilizes blood glucose levels by reducing postprandial hyperglycemia, insulin spikes, and glucose variability associated with high-carbohydrate meals. Lower carbohydrate intake and ketogenic metabolism promote gluconeogenesis, glycogen sparing, and maintenance of euglycemia during fasting or low-energy states, reducing the risk of hypoglycemia and glycemic fluctuations.

- Reduced Risk of Metabolic Disorders: Fat adaptation may reduce the risk of metabolic disorders, such as type 2 diabetes, metabolic syndrome, and cardiovascular diseases, by improving insulin sensitivity, lipid profiles, and inflammatory markers. Lower circulating glucose and insulin levels, coupled with elevated ketone bodies and improved lipid metabolism, contribute to metabolic improvements and cardiometabolic risk reduction in individuals with insulin resistance and obesity.

3. Enhanced Athletic Performance:

- Endurance Adaptations: Fat adaptation enhances endurance performance and exercise capacity by increasing reliance on fat-derived fuels, sparing glycogen stores, and delaying the onset of fatigue during prolonged aerobic activities. Fat-adapted athletes exhibit superior fat oxidation rates, sustained energy levels, and improved metabolic efficiency, translating to enhanced endurance, recovery, and performance outcomes in endurance sports.

- Glycogen Preservation: Fat adaptation preserves glycogen stores and minimizes muscle glycogen depletion during prolonged exercise, allowing athletes to maintain higher intensities and sustain longer durations of aerobic activity without experiencing "bonking" or hitting the wall. Shifts in fuel substrate utilization towards fat oxidation reduce carbohydrate requirements during endurance events, enabling athletes to optimize energy utilization and performance without relying solely on exogenous carbohydrate supplementation.

Practical Strategies for Fat Adaptation and Weight Loss:

1. Carbohydrate Restriction:

- Ketogenic Diet: Adopting a ketogenic diet, characterized by very low carbohydrate intake (<50 grams per day), moderate protein intake, and high fat consumption, induces rapid fat adaptation, ketosis, and metabolic changes conducive to weight loss and metabolic health improvement. Ketogenic diets prioritize whole foods, such as non-starchy vegetables, leafy greens, nuts, seeds, avocados, and healthy fats, while minimizing refined carbohydrates, sugars, and processed foods.

2. Moderate Protein Intake:

- Protein Moderation: Moderate protein intake is essential for fat adaptation and weight loss, as excessive protein consumption may inhibit ketogenesis, gluconeogenesis, and ketone production by stimulating insulin secretion and activating mTOR signaling pathways. Adequate protein intake (0.8-1.2 grams per kilogram of body weight) supports muscle maintenance, satiety signaling, and metabolic health without compromising ketosis or fat oxidation rates.

3. Healthy Fat Sources:

- Nutrient Diverse fat sources are essential for fat adaptation and weight loss, as they provide essential fatty acids, fat-soluble vitamins, and energy substrates for ketogenesis and mitochondrial metabolism. Incorporating a variety of healthy fats into the diet supports metabolic flexibility, satiety, and nutrient adequacy while minimizing inflammation and oxidative stress associated with excessive omega-6 fatty acid intake. Examples of healthy fat sources include:

- Monounsaturated Fats: Foods rich in monounsaturated fats, such as olive oil, avocados, nuts, and seeds, provide heart-healthy fats that support cardiovascular health, insulin sensitivity, and weight management. Monounsaturated fats are associated with reduced risk of metabolic syndrome, type 2 diabetes, and cardiovascular diseases, making them a valuable component of fat-adapted diets.

- Omega-3 Fatty Acids: Omega-3 fatty acids, found in fatty fish (e.g., salmon, mackerel, sardines), flaxseeds, chia seeds, and walnuts, exert anti-inflammatory and cardioprotective effects, improving lipid profiles, endothelial function, and insulin sensitivity. Incorporating omega-3-rich foods into the diet promotes metabolic health, cognitive function, and overall well-being, complementing the fat adaptation process.

- Coconut Products: Coconut products, including coconut oil, coconut milk, and unsweetened shredded coconut, are rich in medium-chain triglycerides (MCTs), which are readily converted into ketone bodies by the liver and used as efficient energy substrates during ketosis. MCTs enhance fat oxidation, thermogenesis, and satiety, supporting weight loss efforts and metabolic health improvements.

- Grass-Fed Butter and Ghee: Grass-fed butter and ghee are excellent sources of conjugated linoleic acid (CLA), vitamin K2, and butyrate, which support metabolic health, gut integrity, and immune function. Grass-fed dairy products contain higher levels of omega-3 fatty acids and fat-soluble vitamins compared to conventional dairy, making them preferable choices for fat adaptation and weight loss.

4. Intermittent Fasting:

- Time-Restricted Eating: Intermittent fasting regimens, such as time-restricted eating (e.g., 16:8 fasting), alternate-day fasting, or periodic fasting, promote fat adaptation, autophagy, and metabolic benefits by restricting the timing of food intake and extending the fasting period between meals. Fasting periods induce metabolic shifts towards fat oxidation, ketogenesis, and cellular repair processes, enhancing weight loss, insulin sensitivity, and longevity.

- Fasting Mimicking Diets: Fasting mimicking diets (FMDs), characterized by low-calorie, plant-based meal plans designed to mimic the physiological effects of fasting while providing essential nutrients and micronutrients, offer an alternative approach for fat adaptation and weight management. FMDs promote metabolic flexibility, cellular rejuvenation, and stress resistance, supporting sustainable weight loss and metabolic improvements without prolonged fasting.

5. Exercise and Physical Activity:

- Resistance Training: Resistance training exercises, such as weightlifting, bodyweight exercises, and resistance band workouts, stimulate muscle growth, increase metabolic rate, and improve insulin sensitivity, contributing to fat loss and lean body mass preservation. Resistance training enhances fat oxidation, mitochondrial biogenesis, and post-exercise energy expenditure, supporting long-term weight management and metabolic health.

- High-Intensity Interval Training (HIIT): High-intensity interval training (HIIT) workouts, characterized by short bursts of intense exercise followed by brief recovery periods, enhance fat adaptation, aerobic capacity, and metabolic efficiency by promoting mitochondrial adaptations, oxidative phosphorylation, and lactate clearance. HIIT sessions improve fat oxidation rates, cardiovascular fitness, and exercise performance, facilitating weight loss and metabolic improvements in individuals with varying fitness levels.

6. Sleep Quality and Stress Management:

- Adequate Sleep: Quality sleep is essential for fat adaptation, weight loss, and metabolic health, as it regulates appetite hormones, such as leptin and ghrelin, and modulates stress responses, cortisol levels, and sympathetic nervous system activity. Prioritizing sleep hygiene practices, such as maintaining a consistent sleep schedule, creating a conducive sleep environment, and minimizing screen time before bedtime, supports optimal sleep duration and quality for metabolic health and weight management.

- Stress Reduction Techniques: Chronic stress disrupts fat metabolism, appetite regulation, and energy balance, contributing to weight gain, visceral adiposity, and metabolic dysfunction. Stress reduction techniques, such as mindfulness meditation, deep breathing exercises, and relaxation therapies, mitigate the impact of stress on fat adaptation, cortisol levels, and inflammatory responses, promoting metabolic resilience and weight loss success.

Fat adaptation offers a promising approach for weight loss and metabolic health improvement, harnessing the body's ability to utilize fats efficiently for energy production, ketone synthesis, and metabolic flexibility. By adopting a low-carbohydrate, high-fat diet, incorporating intermittent fasting, engaging in regular exercise, and prioritizing sleep and stress management, individuals can achieve sustainable weight loss, enhance metabolic health, and optimize overall well-being. Understanding the physiological mechanisms, potential benefits, and practical strategies for fat adaptation empowers individuals to make informed choices that support long-term success in achieving their health and fitness goals. Through personalized approaches, lifestyle modifications, and ongoing support, individuals can embark on a journey towards fat adaptation, weight loss, and metabolic wellness, reclaiming control of their health and vitality.

HUMAN GROWTH HORMONE (HGH) PRODUCTION:

Harnessing the Power of Fasting:

"Is not this the kind of fasting I have chosen: to loose the chains of injustice and untie the cords of the yoke, to set the oppressed free and break every yoke?" - Isaiah 58:6 (NIV)

◆ ◆ ◆

Fasting has been practiced for centuries for spiritual, cultural, and health reasons. In recent years, scientific research has shed light on the physiological effects of fasting, including its impact on hormone regulation. One hormone that has garnered significant attention in relation to fasting is human growth hormone (HGH). This essay explores the intricate relationship between fasting and the increase of human growth hormone production, examining the mechanisms, benefits, and practical implications for health and longevity.

Understanding Human Growth Hormone (HGH):

1. Role in the Body:

   - Growth and Development: Human growth hormone, produced by the pituitary gland, plays a crucial role in growth, development, and maintenance of tissues throughout life. During childhood and adolescence, HGH promotes linear growth, skeletal maturation, and organ development, contributing to height, muscle mass, and bone density.

   - Metabolic Regulation: In addition to its growth-promoting effects, HGH regulates metabolism, energy expenditure, and substrate utilization in adults. HGH stimulates lipolysis, mobilization of fatty acids from adipose tissue, and oxidation of fats for energy production, promoting fat loss and lean body mass preservation.

2. Secretion Patterns:

   - Pulsatile Release: HGH secretion occurs in a pulsatile manner, with peaks and troughs throughout the day in response to various stimuli, including sleep, exercise, stress, and nutrient intake. The largest pulse of HGH secretion typically occurs shortly after the onset of deep sleep, during the early stages of the nocturnal sleep cycle.

- Age-Related Decline: HGH secretion declines with age, peaking during childhood and adolescence and gradually declining thereafter. By adulthood, HGH levels decrease significantly, contributing to age-related changes in body composition, metabolism, and physical function.

Mechanisms of HGH Regulation During Fasting:

1. Growth Hormone-Releasing Hormone (GHRH) and Growth Hormone-Inhibiting Hormone (GHIH):

- Hypothalamic Regulation: HGH secretion is regulated by a complex interplay of hypothalamic hormones, including growth hormone-releasing hormone (GHRH) and growth hormone-inhibiting hormone (GHIH), also known as somatostatin. GHRH stimulates HGH synthesis and release from the pituitary gland, whereas GHIH inhibits HGH secretion.

2. Nutrient Sensing Pathways:

- Insulin-Like Growth Factor-1 (IGF-1): Insulin-like growth factor-1 (IGF-1), a key mediator of HGH actions, regulates HGH secretion through negative feedback mechanisms. High levels of circulating glucose and insulin suppress HGH secretion by increasing IGF-1 production, whereas low levels of glucose and insulin, as seen during fasting, stimulate HGH release.

- Glucose Availability: Glucose availability plays a crucial role in modulating HGH secretion during fasting. Reduced glucose levels, coupled with increased fatty acid oxidation and ketone production, signal the body to upregulate HGH production as a compensatory mechanism to preserve lean body mass, mobilize stored energy reserves, and promote metabolic adaptation to fasting.

- Amino Acid Levels: Amino acids, particularly arginine and lysine, stimulate HGH secretion through direct effects on the pituitary gland and hypothalamus. Fasting-induced amino acid depletion, followed by refeeding or protein ingestion, triggers a transient increase in HGH secretion, known as the "protein-sparing effect," which facilitates protein synthesis and tissue repair.

Benefits of Increased HGH Production During Fasting:

1. Enhanced Fat Metabolism:

- Lipolysis and Fat Oxidation: Increased HGH

secretion during fasting promotes lipolysis, the breakdown of triglycerides into fatty acids and glycerol, and fat oxidation, the utilization of fatty acids for energy production. Elevated HGH levels enhance adipose tissue lipolysis, mobilization of stored fats, and oxidation of fatty acids in skeletal muscle, liver, and other tissues, facilitating fat loss and body composition improvements.

- Reduction of Visceral Fat: Fasting-induced HGH release targets visceral adipose tissue, the "dangerous" fat stored around organs, which is associated with increased risk of metabolic disorders, cardiovascular diseases, and insulin resistance. By promoting preferential mobilization and oxidation of visceral fat stores, HGH contributes to reductions in abdominal obesity and improvements in metabolic health markers.

2. Preservation of Lean Body Mass:

- Protein Sparing Effect: HGH exerts a protein-sparing effect during fasting by promoting the preservation of lean body mass, including skeletal muscle, organs, and structural proteins. Increased HGH levels stimulate protein synthesis, nitrogen retention, and tissue repair processes, while inhibiting protein breakdown and catabolism, thereby preserving muscle mass and functional integrity during periods of energy restriction.

- Anabolic Effects: HGH enhances the anabolic effects of other hormones, such as testosterone and insulin, by promoting amino acid uptake, protein synthesis, and cell growth in muscle tissue. By synergizing with insulin and testosterone, HGH facilitates muscle hypertrophy, strength gains, and physical performance improvements, supporting muscle maintenance and adaptation to fasting-induced metabolic stress.

3. Metabolic Adaptation and Longevity:

- Metabolic Flexibility: Fasting-induced HGH release promotes metabolic flexibility, the ability of the body to switch between different fuel sources, including glucose and fatty acids, in response to changes in nutrient availability and energy demands - Hormonal Regulation: Fasting-induced increases in HGH levels contribute to hormonal adaptations that optimize energy metabolism, insulin sensitivity, and oxidative stress resistance, promoting metabolic health and longevity. HGH interacts with other hormones, such as insulin, glucagon, and cortisol, to regulate glucose homeostasis, ketogenesis, and lipid metabolism, ensuring energy balance and metabolic stability during fasting periods.

4. Cellular Repair and Regeneration:

- Tissue Regeneration: Elevated HGH levels during fasting stimulate tissue repair, regeneration, and rejuvenation processes, including wound healing, cellular proliferation, and stem cell activation. HGH promotes tissue remodeling, collagen synthesis, and angiogenesis, facilitating the repair of damaged tissues, organs, and skin, while enhancing resilience to oxidative stress and environmental toxins.

- Autophagy Induction: Fasting-induced HGH release triggers autophagy, a cellular recycling process that removes damaged organelles, protein aggregates, and dysfunctional components, promoting cellular detoxification and renewal. HGH-mediated activation of autophagy pathways enhances cellular quality control mechanisms, mitochondrial function, and longevity pathways, contributing to cellular homeostasis and stress resistance.

Practical Implications of Fasting for Increasing HGH Levels:

1. Intermittent Fasting Protocols:

- Time-Restricted Eating: Adopt time-restricted eating patterns, such as the 16:8 fasting protocol, which involves fasting for 16 hours and limiting food intake to an 8-hour feeding window. Time-restricted eating aligns with natural circadian rhythms and promotes HGH secretion during the overnight fasting period, maximizing the benefits of fasting-induced hormonal responses.

- Alternate-Day Fasting: Implement alternate-day fasting regimens, alternating between fasting days and ad libitum eating days, to induce periodic increases in HGH levels and metabolic adaptations. Alternate-day fasting promotes metabolic flexibility, fat loss, and autophagy activation, while supporting muscle preservation and cellular rejuvenation during fasting periods.

2. Extended Fasting:

- Periodic Fasting: Incorporate periodic fasting protocols, such as multi-day water fasts or prolonged fasting mimicking diets, to induce deeper metabolic adaptations, stem cell activation, and systemic rejuvenation. Extended fasting periods of 24-72 hours stimulate robust increases in HGH secretion, autophagy induction, and cellular repair processes, supporting metabolic reset and longevity enhancement.

- Supervised Fasting: Consider supervised fasting programs conducted under medical supervision, particularly for individuals with underlying health conditions or medication regimens. Supervised fasting protocols provide guidance, monitoring, and support to ensure safety, efficacy, and optimal outcomes, while minimizing potential risks associated with prolonged fasting.

3. Nutritional Considerations:

- Optimize Nutrient Intake: Prioritize nutrient-dense foods, such as lean proteins, healthy fats, fibrous vegetables, and micronutrient-rich foods, during feeding periods to support metabolic health, muscle maintenance, and hormonal balance. Adequate intake of essential nutrients, including amino acids, vitamins, and minerals, is essential for HGH synthesis, secretion, and biological activity.

- Replenish Electrolytes: Maintain electrolyte balance during fasting periods by consuming electrolyte-rich fluids, such as water with added electrolyte supplements or bone broth, to prevent dehydration, electrolyte imbalances, and adverse symptoms associated with fasting, such as fatigue, dizziness, or muscle cramps.

Fasting represents a powerful tool for increasing human growth hormone (HGH) production, promoting metabolic health, and enhancing longevity. By inducing transient increases in HGH secretion, fasting activates cellular repair mechanisms, enhances fat metabolism, preserves lean body mass, and supports metabolic adaptation to energy restriction. Through strategic implementation of intermittent fasting protocols, extended fasting regimens, and nutritional optimization strategies, individuals can harness the benefits of fasting-induced HGH release to optimize healthspan and promote longevity. However, it's important to approach fasting with caution, especially for individuals with medical conditions or specific dietary needs, and to seek guidance from healthcare professionals when incorporating fasting into a lifestyle routine. With mindful application and personalized adjustments, fasting can serve as a valuable tool for optimizing hormonal balance, metabolic resilience, and overall well-being throughout the lifespan.

REDUCED CARBOHYDRATE AND LONGEVITY:

Exploring Mechanisms, Benefits, and Practical Implications

◆ ◆ ◆

In recent years, the relationship between dietary patterns and longevity has garnered significant attention from researchers and health enthusiasts alike. Among various dietary approaches, reducing carbohydrate intake has emerged as a promising strategy for promoting longevity and improving overall health span. This chapter aims to delve into the connection between reduced carbohydrate intake and longevity, examining the underlying mechanisms, potential benefits, and practical implications for enhancing longevity and optimizing health.

Understanding Reduced Carbohydrate Intake:

1. Definition and Rationale:

- Reduced carbohydrate intake involves limiting the consumption of carbohydrates, particularly refined sugars and starches, in favor of protein, healthy fats, and non-starchy vegetables. This dietary approach prioritizes nutrient-dense foods while minimizing the insulinogenic and glycemic effects of high-carbohydrate meals, promoting metabolic flexibility, weight management, and longevity.

- Rationale: The rationale behind reducing carbohydrate intake stems from the adverse health effects associated with excessive carbohydrate consumption, including insulin resistance, obesity, inflammation, and chronic diseases. By moderating carbohydrate intake, individuals can mitigate these risks, optimize metabolic health, and potentially extend lifespan by reducing the burden of metabolic dysfunction and age-related diseases.

2. Types of Reduced Carbohydrate Diets:

- Ketogenic Diet: The ketogenic diet is a low-carbohydrate, high-fat diet that induces nutritional ketosis, a metabolic state characterized by elevated ketone levels and increased fat oxidation. Ketogenic diets typically restrict carbohydrate intake to less than 50 grams per day, promoting ketogenesis, ketone utilization, and metabolic adaptations conducive to longevity and healthspan extension.

- Low-Carbohydrate Diet: Low-carbohydrate diets encompass a spectrum of carbohydrate intake levels, ranging from moderate carbohydrate restriction (e.g., 50-150 grams per day) to very low-carbohydrate intake (<50 grams per day). These diets prioritize whole foods, fibrous vegetables, lean proteins, and healthy fats while minimizing processed carbohydrates, sugars, and refined grains.

Mechanisms Underlying Reduced Carbohydrate Intake and Longevity:

1. Metabolic Benefits:

- Enhanced Insulin Sensitivity: Reduced carbohydrate intake improves insulin sensitivity and glucose metabolism by minimizing postprandial glycemic excursions, reducing insulin secretion, and promoting cellular glucose uptake. Lower carbohydrate diets attenuate hyperinsulinemia, insulin resistance, and inflammation, mitigating the risk of metabolic disorders associated with carbohydrate-rich diets.

- Ketone Metabolism: Ketogenic diets promote the production of ketone bodies, such as beta-hydroxybutyrate (BHB), acetoacetate, and acetone, which serve as alternative energy substrates for tissues, including the brain, heart, and skeletal muscle. Ketones enhance mitochondrial efficiency, oxidative stress resistance, and cellular repair mechanisms, supporting longevity and healthspan extension.

2. Hormonal Regulation:

- Growth Hormone and IGF-1: Reduced carbohydrate intake modulates growth hormone (GH) and insulin-like growth factor-1 (IGF-1) signaling pathways, promoting metabolic adaptations, cellular repair processes, and longevity-associated gene expression patterns. Lower insulin and IGF-1 levels, coupled with increased GH secretion, enhance autophagy, DNA repair, and stress resistance mechanisms implicated in longevity and aging.

- Sirtuin Activation: Sirtuins, a family of NAD +-dependent protein deacetylases, play a critical role in regulating cellular metabolism, oxidative stress responses, and longevity pathways. Reduced carbohydrate intake activates sirtuin enzymes, such as SIRT1 and SIRT3, which promote mitochondrial biogenesis, DNA repair, and antioxidant defenses, enhancing cellular resilience and longevity potential.

3. Inflammatory Modulation:

- Reduction of Chronic Inflammation: Excessive carbohydrate consumption contributes to chronic low-grade inflammation, oxidative stress, and immune dysregulation, driving the pathogenesis of age-related diseases, such as cardiovascular diseases, neurodegenerative disorders, and cancer. By reducing carbohydrate intake, individuals can attenuate inflammatory cytokine production, NF-kB activation, and pro-inflammatory signaling pathways implicated in aging and age-related morbidity.

- Anti-inflammatory Effects of Ketones: Ketone bodies exhibit anti-inflammatory properties by inhibiting NLRP3 inflammasome activation, reducing reactive oxygen species (ROS) production, and modulating immune cell function. Beta-hydroxybutyrate (BHB) acts as a histone deacetylase (HDAC) inhibitor, suppressing pro-inflammatory gene expression and promoting a state of metabolic and immune quiescence conducive to longevity and healthspan extension.

Benefits of Reduced Carbohydrate Intake for Longevity:

1. Weight Management:

- Fat Loss and Body Composition: Reduced carbohydrate intake promotes fat loss, preservation of lean muscle mass, and improvements in body composition by enhancing fat oxidation, suppressing appetite, and promoting satiety signaling. Ketogenic diets induce rapid weight loss, particularly visceral adiposity, by mobilizing stored fat reserves for energy production and supporting metabolic adaptations conducive to fat metabolism.

- Metabolic Health: Lower carbohydrate diets improve metabolic health parameters, such as insulin sensitivity, blood lipid profiles, and inflammatory markers, reducing the risk of obesity-related comorbidities, such as type 2 diabetes, cardiovascular diseases, and non-alcoholic fatty liver disease (NAFLD). By optimizing metabolic function, individuals can enhance longevity potential and reduce the burden of age-related metabolic disorders.

2. Cognitive Function:

- Neuroprotective Effects: Reduced carbohydrate intake and ketogenic metabolism exert neuroprotective effects by enhancing mitochondrial function, synaptic plasticity, and neuronal resilience against oxidative stress and excitotoxicity. Ketone bodies serve as efficient energy substrates for the brain, supporting cognitive function, memory consolidation, and neurotransmitter synthesis, while mitigating age-related cognitive decline and neurodegenerative diseases.

- Alzheimer's Disease Prevention: Emerging evidence suggests that reduced carbohydrate intake and ketone metabolism may offer therapeutic benefits for Alzheimer's disease prevention and treatment by improving cerebral energy metabolism, reducing amyloid-beta accumulation, and modulating neuroinflammatory pathways. Ketogenic diets and exogenous ketone supplementation hold promise for preserving cognitive function and delaying disease progression in individuals at risk for Alzheimer's disease.

3. Cardiovascular Health:

- Improved Lipid Profiles: Reduced carbohydrate diets improve blood lipid profiles by increasing high-density lipoprotein (HDL) cholesterol levels, reducing triglycerides, and shifting the LDL particle distribution towards larger, less atherogenic particles. Favorable changes in lipid metabolism, such as increased HDL-to-LDL ratio and decreased triglyceride-to-HDL ratio, reduce the risk of atherosclerosis, coronary artery disease, and cardiovascular events.

- Blood Pressure Regulation: Ketogenic diets and reduced carbohydrate intake may lower blood pressure and improve vascular function by reducing insulin levels, enhancing nitric oxide bioavailability, and promoting endothelial health. Improved blood pressure control and arterial compliance contribute to cardiovascular health, reducing the risk of hypertension, stroke, and peripheral vascular diseases associated with aging and metabolic dysfunction.

Practical Implications of Reduced Carbohydrate Intake for Longevity:

1. Dietary Strategies:

- Whole Foods Emphasis: Prioritize nutrient-dense, whole foods, including non-starchy vegetables, leafy greens, lean proteins, healthy fats, and nuts/seeds, while minimizing processed carbohydrates, sugars, and refined grains. Emphasize variety, freshness, and quality in food choices to maximize nutrient intake and promote metabolic health.

- Carbohydrate Restriction: Reduce consumption of high-glycemic carbohydrates, such as sugar, white bread, pasta, and pastries, in favor of low-glycemic options, such as whole grains, legumes, and fibrous vegetables. Aim to consume carbohydrates primarily from non-starchy vegetables, berries, and moderate portions of whole grains to support metabolic flexibility and blood sugar regulation.

- Ketogenic Diet: Consider adopting a ketogenic diet, characterized by very low carbohydrate intake (<50 grams per day), moderate protein consumption, and high fat intake. Prioritize healthy sources of fats, such as avocado, olive oil, nuts, seeds, and fatty fish, while incorporating small amounts of low-carbohydrate vegetables and protein-rich foods to meet nutrient needs and maintain satiety.

2. Intermittent Fasting:

- Time-Restricted Eating: Implement time-restricted eating (e.g., 16:8 fasting) to restrict the window of food consumption and extend the fasting period between meals. Gradually increase fasting duration and experiment with different fasting protocols to identify an approach that suits individual preferences, lifestyle, and metabolic goals.

- Periodic Fasting: Explore periodic fasting regimens, such as alternate-day fasting, 5:2 fasting, or extended fasting, to challenge metabolic flexibility, promote autophagy, and induce cellular repair mechanisms associated with longevity and healthspan extension. Consult with a healthcare professional before embarking on prolonged fasting protocols, particularly for individuals with underlying health conditions or medication regimens.

3. Lifestyle Modifications:

- Regular Physical Activity: Engage in regular physical activity, including aerobic exercise, resistance training, and flexibility exercises, to support metabolic health, cardiovascular fitness, and musculoskeletal function. Incorporate both structured exercise sessions and daily movement activities, such as walking, cycling, or gardening, to maintain an active lifestyle and enhance longevity.

- Stress Management: Practice stress reduction techniques, such as mindfulness meditation, deep breathing exercises, and relaxation therapies, to mitigate the impact of chronic stress on metabolic health, immune function, and aging processes. Cultivate resilience, positive coping strategies, and social support networks to buffer against stressors and promote emotional well-being.

- Quality Sleep: Prioritize quality sleep hygiene practices, such as maintaining a consistent sleep schedule, creating a conducive sleep environment, and practicing relaxation rituals before bedtime, to optimize sleep duration and quality. Aim for 7-9 hours of restorative sleep per night to support cellular repair, cognitive function, and hormonal balance essential for longevity.

4. Personalized Approach:

- Individualized Assessment: Tailor dietary and lifestyle interventions to individual needs, preferences, and metabolic profiles by conducting personalized assessments, such as metabolic testing, genetic analysis, and medical evaluations. Consult with qualified healthcare professionals, including registered dietitians, nutritionists, and physicians, to develop personalized plans based on comprehensive assessments and health goals.

- Monitoring and Adjustments: Monitor biomarkers, health indicators, and subjective measures of well-being to track progress, identify areas for improvement, and make informed adjustments to dietary and lifestyle strategies. Regularly reassess goals, modify interventions as needed, and celebrate milestones to maintain motivation and momentum towards achieving longevity and optimal health.

Reducing carbohydrate intake holds promise as a dietary strategy for promoting longevity, optimizing metabolic health, and enhancing overall well-being. By prioritizing nutrient-dense foods, minimizing processed carbohydrates, and incorporating intermittent fasting and lifestyle modifications, individuals can support metabolic flexibility, reduce the risk of age-related diseases, and extend health span. Through personalized approaches, ongoing self-assessment, and collaborative support from healthcare professionals, individuals can embark on a journey towards longevity and vitality, enjoying the benefits of optimized health and quality of life for years to come.

UNLEASHING BOUNDLESS ENERGY:

Exploring the Keto Diet's Impact on Energy Levels

"Food addiction is not about weakness; it's about biochemistry."

◆ ◆ ◆

In recent years, the ketogenic diet (keto diet) has gained widespread popularity for its potential to not only aid in weight loss but also for its purported ability to enhance energy levels and promote vitality. By drastically reducing carbohydrate intake and increasing fat consumption, the keto diet shifts the body's primary fuel source from glucose to ketones, which are derived from fat metabolism. This chapter delves into the intricate relationship between the keto diet and energy, examining the physiological mechanisms, practical implications, and potential benefits for optimizing energy levels and overall well-being.

Understanding the Keto Diet and Energy Metabolism:

1. Overview of the Keto Diet:

- The ketogenic diet is a high-fat, moderate-protein, and low-carbohydrate dietary approach designed to induce nutritional ketosis, a metabolic state characterized by elevated ketone bodies in the bloodstream. By restricting carbohydrate intake to a minimal level (typically less than 50 grams per day) and increasing fat consumption, the keto diet promotes a shift in energy metabolism from glucose to ketones for fuel.

- Ketogenic Macros: The keto diet typically consists of macronutrient ratios that prioritize fat intake (approximately 70-80% of total calories), followed by moderate protein consumption (approximately 20-25% of total calories), and minimal carbohydrate intake (approximately 5-10% of total calories). This macronutrient distribution aims to induce and sustain ketosis, a metabolic state associated with increased fat oxidation and ketone production.

2. Energy Metabolism on the Keto Diet:
- Glucose vs. Ketones: In a standard

Western diet rich in carbohydrates, the body primarily relies on glucose derived from dietary carbohydrates for energy production. However, in a ketogenic state induced by the keto diet, the body transitions to utilizing ketones, produced from fatty acids via hepatic ketogenesis, as its primary fuel source. Ketones, such as beta-hydroxybutyrate (BHB), acetoacetate, and acetone, are efficiently utilized by the brain, heart, muscles, and other tissues for energy production.

- Metabolic Adaptations: During the initial stages of transitioning to a ketogenic state, the body undergoes metabolic adaptations to optimize ketone utilization and energy production. Liver glycogen stores are depleted, insulin levels decrease, and ketone production increases, facilitating the transition from glucose to fat metabolism. As ketosis is established, the body becomes increasingly efficient at mobilizing and oxidizing fatty acids for energy, leading to sustained ketone production and enhanced energy levels.

Physiological Mechanisms Behind Increased Energy on the Keto Diet:

1. Enhanced Fat Oxidation:

- Efficient Fuel Source: Ketones derived from fat metabolism serve as a highly efficient fuel source for cellular energy production, particularly in tissues with high metabolic demands, such as the brain, heart, and skeletal muscles. Unlike glucose, which requires insulin for cellular uptake, ketones can freely cross the blood-brain barrier and enter mitochondria for oxidation, providing a steady supply of energy without fluctuations in blood sugar levels.

- Mitochondrial Efficiency: Ketogenic metabolism enhances mitochondrial efficiency and oxidative capacity, promoting mitochondrial biogenesis, ATP production, and electron transport chain function. By optimizing mitochondrial function, the keto diet increases cellular energy output, reduces oxidative stress, and enhances endurance and physical performance, contributing to sustained energy levels and vitality.

2. Stable Blood Sugar Levels:

- Glycemic Control: The keto diet promotes stable blood sugar levels and mitigates fluctuations in insulin and glucose, which are common triggers for energy crashes and fatigue on high-carbohydrate diets. By minimizing carbohydrate intake and moderating insulin secretion, the keto diet helps regulate blood sugar levels, preventing energy spikes and crashes associated with glycemic variability.

- Reduced Glycogen Depletion: Unlike

carbohydrate-dependent metabolism, which relies on glycogen stores for energy during periods of fasting or exercise, ketogenic metabolism prioritizes fat oxidation and ketone utilization, sparing glycogen reserves for high-intensity activities and metabolic demands. By preserving glycogen stores and promoting fat adaptation, the keto diet supports sustained energy levels and metabolic flexibility across varying energy requirements.

3. Brain Health and Cognitive Function:

- Neurological Benefits: Ketones produced during ketosis have neuroprotective properties and provide an alternative energy source for the brain, supporting cognitive function, mood regulation, and mental clarity. Beta-hydroxybutyrate (BHB), the primary circulating ketone, enhances synaptic plasticity, neurotransmitter balance, and mitochondrial function in neurons, promoting cognitive resilience and focus on the keto diet.

- Mental Clarity: Many individuals report experiencing improved mental clarity, heightened focus, and sustained energy levels on the keto diet, attributed to the stable supply of ketones to the brain and reduced reliance on glucose for energy. By reducing brain fog, enhancing cognitive performance, and supporting mood stability, the keto diet contributes to overall well-being and productivity.

Practical Implications and Tips for Optimizing Energy on the Keto Diet:

1. Adequate Fat Intake:

- Quality Fats: Prioritize healthy sources of fats, such as avocados, olive oil, nuts, seeds, and fatty fish, to meet daily fat requirements and support ketosis. Include a variety of monounsaturated, polyunsaturated, and saturated fats in the diet to ensure optimal nutrient intake and metabolic flexibility.

- Medium-Chain Triglycerides (MCTs): Incorporate MCT oil or coconut oil into meals and beverages to boost ketone production, enhance fat oxidation, and support energy levels. MCTs are rapidly absorbed and converted into ketones by the liver, providing a quick and sustained source of energy during fasting or physical activity.

2. Moderate Protein Consumption:

- Lean Proteins: Consume moderate amounts of high-quality protein sources, such as poultry, fish, eggs, and tofu, to support muscle maintenance, satiety, and metabolic function. Avoid excessive protein intake, which can interfere with ketosis by promoting gluconeogenesis and insulin secretion.

3. Electrolyte Balance:

- Sodium, Potassium, Magnesium: Maintain electrolyte balance by supplementing with sodium, potassium, and magnesium to prevent electrolyte imbalances, dehydration, and fatigue associated with the keto flu. Include electrolyte-rich foods, such as leafy greens, avocado, and bone broth, in the diet to support hydration and mineral balance.

4. Hydration:

- Water Intake: Stay adequately hydrated by drinking water throughout the day, especially during fasting periods or in hot climates. Adequate hydration supports cellular function, metabolism, and energy production, while preventing dehydration-related fatigue and cognitive impairment.

5. Listen to Your Body:

- Individual Variation: Pay attention to your body's signals and adjust your dietary approach based on individual needs, preferences, and energy requirements. Experiment with different meal timings, macronutrient ratios, and fasting protocols to find the optimal balance for sustained energy levels and well-being.

The ketogenic diet offers a unique approach to enhancing energy levels, optimizing metabolic function, and promoting overall well-being through the metabolic adaptation to ketosis. By prioritizing fat metabolism, stabilizing blood sugar levels, and supporting brain health, the keto diet provides a sustainable source of energy for both physical and cognitive performance. By understanding the physiological mechanisms behind increased energy on the keto diet and implementing practical strategies for optimizing energy levels, individuals can unlock boundless vitality, mental clarity, and metabolic resilience on their journey towards optimal health and wellness.

Here are 7 anonymous quotes about food addiction.

1. "Food addiction is real, and it's time we treat it with the seriousness it deserves."

2. "Just like any other addiction, food addiction can consume your thoughts, emotions, and actions."

3. "Food addiction doesn't discriminate; it affects people of all ages, backgrounds, and walks of life."

4. "Breaking free from food addiction requires more than willpower; it demands understanding, support, and compassion."

5. "Food addiction is not a character flaw; it's a complex interplay of genetics, environment, and neurobiology."

6. "In a world where food is abundant and temptation is everywhere, overcoming food addiction is a daily battle for many."

7. "Food addiction can feel like a prison, but recovery is possible with courage, determination, and the right tools."

Here are 8 anonymous quotes about fasting:

1. "Fasting is the body's way of resetting, rejuvenating, and renewing itself from the inside out."

2. "In the stillness of fasting, the body finds healing, the mind finds clarity, and the spirit finds peace."

3. "Fasting is not about deprivation; it's about liberation from the chains of excess and the burdens of overconsumption."

4. "Through fasting, we discover the power of restraint, the resilience of the human body, and the depths of our inner strength."

5. "Fasting is a journey inward, where we

confront our fears, cravings, and attachments, and emerge lighter, stronger, and more aligned with our true selves."

6. "In the absence of food, we find sustenance in silence, solace in simplicity, and strength in surrender."

7. "Fasting teaches us patience, discipline, and gratitude for the abundance that surrounds us."

8. "Fasting is not a punishment for the body; it's a gift of healing, renewal, and regeneration.

Here are 10 biblical quotes regarding fasting.

1. "But when you fast, put oil on your head and wash your face, so that it will not be obvious to others that you are fasting, but only to your Father, who is unseen; and your Father, who sees what is done in secret, will reward you." - Matthew 6:17-18 (NIV)

2. "Is not this the kind of fasting I have chosen: to loose the chains of injustice and untie the cords of the yoke, to set the oppressed free and break every yoke?" - Isaiah 58:6 (NIV)

3. "So we fasted and petitioned our God about this, and he answered our prayer." - Ezra 8:23 (NIV)

4. "But I, when they were ill— I put on sackcloth and humbled myself with fasting. When my prayers returned to me unanswered," - Psalm 35:13 (NIV)

5. "After fasting forty days and forty nights, he was hungry." - Matthew 4:2 (NIV)

6. "So after they had fasted and prayed, they placed their hands on them and sent them off." - Acts 13:3 (NIV)

7. "And Cornelius said, 'Four days ago I was fasting until this hour; and at the ninth hour I prayed in my house, and behold, a man stood before me in bright clothing.'" - Acts 10:30 (NIV)

8. "And he said to them, 'This kind cannot be driven out by anything but prayer and fasting.'" - Mark 9:29 (NIV)

9. "Go, gather together all the Jews who are in Susa, and fast for me. Do not eat or drink for three days, night or day. I and my attendants will fast as you do. When this is done, I will go to the king, even though it is against the law. And if I perish, I perish." - Esther 4:16 (NIV)

10. "So we fasted and petitioned our God about this, and he answered our prayer." - Ezra 8:23 (NIV)

AFTERWORD

ABOUT THE AUTHOR

Zachary Scott Turnage

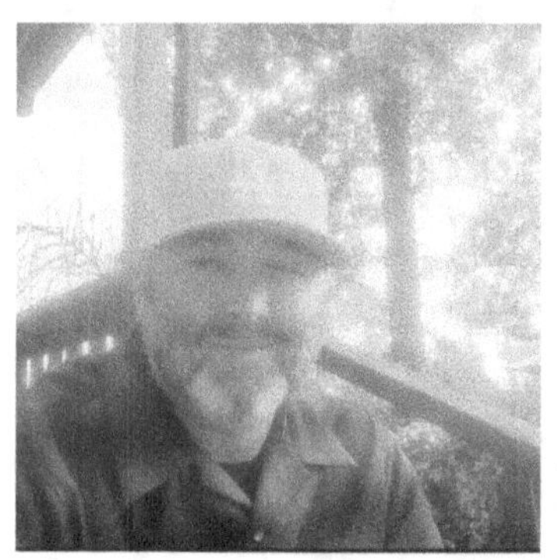

Growing up in the rough streets of Los Angeles Harbor and raised by a single parent on limited income, I truly know the meaning of "The Struggle Is Real". One of the most important lessons I ever learned is that it does not matter where you come from or how you were raised. What does matter is discipline and the drive you carry within you to overcome adversity. Now I enjoy the life of a self-made entrepreneur in stark contrast to being homeless, broke and living in my car several years ago. I am here to tell you that your dreams and destiny awaits your decision to act.

PRAISE FOR AUTHOR

5.0 out of 5 stars Having Courage
Reviewed in the United States on January 13, 2024
A book of courage in faith. Very inspirational. A book of hope. A personal story that can be related too.

- COURAGEMILL

Teresa Jellison
5.0 out of 5 stars the measure of a writer
Reviewed in the United States on February 25, 2024
Verified Purchase
1. When a story grabs the reader in the first sentence and the reader reluctantly allows release at the end
2. Readers know authenticity. This story is written with complete candor, honesty, and courage from genuine experience
3. The last page is reluctantly turned leaving the reader hungry for more

- MOSAIC OF MERCY

Amazon Customer
5.0 out of 5 stars Having Courage
Reviewed in the United States on January 13, 2024
A book of courage in faith. Very inspirational. A book of hope. A personal story that can be related too.

- COURAGEMILL

Lindsay A. McIntyre
5.0 out of 5 stars Powerful!
Reviewed in the United States on December 30, 2023
Verified Purchase
This book is one you will read and re-read! The message of understanding resentment and anger and how it relates to living a forgiving lifestyle are well thought out challenged me to think in ways I didn't know I needed. Much needed!

- MOSAIC OF MERCY